DISCLAIMER

I am not a doctor, nor do I have medical training. I am, however, deeply invested in your health and happiness. I am not a therapist, but I care very much about helping you feel great about yourself. Lastly, I am not a dermatologist, yet this book will offer you valuable, tested ways to help heal your skin. This book conveys everything I've learned from self-experimentation. While the methods in the book are natural and gentle, always proceed with caution. If you have even the smallest health issues, always check with your doctor first. Your health and safety are extremely important to me.

YOU CAN'T
HIDE YOUR FACE

A natural guide to healing acne & loving your skin.

Katherine Larsen
CHC, IAHC, AADP

To contact the author, visit
www.crazyforliving.com

ISBN: 0996155104
ISBN-13: 978-0996155106

DEDICATION

I dedicate this book to all of my readers who are struggling with skin issues. You are the reason for this book. My hope for you is that my journey will help you heal quickly and more gracefully than I did. May you find immediate comfort in knowing that you're not alone.

CONTENTS

ACKNOWLEDGMENTS

Gratitude is everything and I am grateful beyond words for the amazing support I received throughout this process and in my life. Many small moments and kind actions have contributed to making this book a reality. I am thankful for everyone who has ever had a positive impact on me or encouraged me in any way. I would especially like to thank the following people for their contributions:

Josie Kranz - Without your crazy idea, I would not have started, so I can't thank you enough!

Brenda Potter - Thank you for always being there with your incredible healing gifts.

Ian Potter - Thank you for your infectious joy and wonderful spirit.

Lina Yang - Thank you for helping me through challenging skin issues, trusting me, and being so flexible with your approach.

Sue Dwiggins - For always coming to my rescue with an essential oil and a remedy, thank you.

Sue Gilad - Thank you for your incredible guidance and feedback.

Kelly Suzan Waggoner - I am grateful for your amazing talent and making this book come together so quickly!

Carol Jenkins - Thank you for being so flexible, fast and wonderful to work with under such a short time frame.

Jenna Lee Barber - For all of the beautiful and tender support and for always keeping me healthy, thank you.

Cate Nielsen - Thank you for your tireless photography and beautiful editing.

Stephanie Shaner - Your spirit and authenticity is so beautiful and I cannot thank you enough for your many contributions to this book. I can't wait to see what you'll do next!

David Shaner - Thanks for all of the great advice and many long discussions.

Johanna Boberg - Thank you for the ongoing encouragement and always making sure I had healthy and delicious food to keep me going! I am so grateful to have you as a talented mentor and wonderful friend.

Wade Durham - Thank you for your uplifting positivity, your love of music and for all the laughs!

Steven Norton - You are like a bright light that lifts me up exactly when I need it most. Thank you.

Neal and Hannah Chapman - Thank you for the touching feedback on my personal healing story that helped to get this book started.

Dayna Thompson - Thank you for believing in me since day one. You are like a big sister to me.

To Sharon Hyde, Travis Hyde, and Ellie - Thank you for all of the love, support, and mostly for just being you. Spending time at the Hyde farm always feels like home.

Lisa Arnold and the entire Arnold family - Thank you for always being there, even so many miles away. Lisa, thank you so much for your limitless belief in me.

Wayne Hall - Thank you for your constant support, patience, and limitless knowledge. You have helped me in countless ways.

To my UHS family - So many of you have played a big role in my life and have believed in me from day one. I have been incredibly blessed for the wonderful mentors and lifelong friends I have made there. Thank you all from the bottom of my heart.

Thank you so much to my clients, family, and friends who have asked for advice, recipes, and remedies. Your faith in me has provided a wealth of knowledge that continues to help others get well. That means more to me than anything.

A special thanks to my family for making me who I am today.

Dad - I am forever grateful for the incredible work ethic and kind nature that you modeled for me. Please take a vacation soon!

Mom - My comfort is knowing that you will always be there with love and support, no matter what.

David - Your genuine nature is inspiring and your energy contagious. I am so proud to be your sister.

To my amazing and courageous health coaching clients - Your progress inspires me every day and I couldn't be more proud of you!

To my wonderful friends, mentors, and the entire Institute for Integrative Nutrition community - I am so grateful and blessed to know all of you! You have helped me in so many ways and I couldn't have done it without you. Thanks for your belief in me and for the encouragement and constant support. It really does take a village!

To the incredible online health community and everyone listed in my Resource Guide - I have eternal gratitude for the amazing work of every author, researcher, experimenter, biohacker, food blogger, and DIY recipe creator out there. Your hard work contributed an incredible amount to my healing. Our growth is proportionate to our open minds.

PREFACE

Adult acne is not something I ever expected to face. I'd never had skin problems, not even as a teenager, and never thought that I might, one day, suffer from acne as an adult. Pimples, blemishes and outbreaks seemed to be something that I simply didn't have to deal with. I figured it wasn't in my genes and I took my clear skin for granted. I thought my skin would stay great forever, especially since I had invested in facials and expensive skin care products.

So when I went to bed one night as a twenty-five year old woman with clear, vibrant skin, I never imagined that I'd wake up with acne. But I did. Everywhere. There must have been at least fifty pimples protruding from my face. I pressed close to the mirror to examine each one. I prodded them lightly, confusion stricken. What is happening? Literally, overnight, I developed adult acne that covered my entire face. I will never forget that feeling of staring into the mirror and not recognizing myself.

From there, the pimples quickly developed into painful cystic acne, blackheads, whiteheads—you name it, I had it. No part of my face remained clear. No matter what I did, I couldn't rid my skin of this new curse. Acne had invaded my life and instantly changed how I faced the world.

I spent the next five years trying to get rid of my acne, and it got much worse before it got better. I tried every cleanser, acne treatment, and detox diet I could find. Every morning, I painfully inspected my face and applied lots of makeup, trying desperately to hide. A demanding career in the corporate world made my skin issues even more problematic. How could anyone take me seriously when I had the face of a teenager?

Even worse than others judging me, I noticed a change in my own attitude. My confidence severely suffered. I stayed home more.

I canceled plans with friends. I was miserable. Through a long journey and much frustration, my skin only started to heal when I came to accept that everything I thought I knew about skin care was wrong.

I share with you my personal journey through the confusing and embarrassing struggle of acne in the hopes that it helps you to find your healing more easily and more quickly than I did. It wasn't until I changed my diet, ditched my expensive chemical products, managed my stress, and dramatically changed my overall relationship with my skin that it finally began to clear and ultimately heal.

This book is meant to be a resource for all of you who are facing the detrimental challenge of trying to heal your skin. This book is not about topical acne treatments. It is not about telling you not to touch your face, or to take a pill for your hormones, or to just wash your face more. It is not about telling you it's your age or that you just have to suffer through it. What all of the skincare brands, marketing geniuses, and beauty experts might not tell you is that healing your skin comes from the inside out. When you truly nourish your body and your mind, your skin will follow.

My story begins with my healing.

1

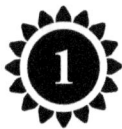

My Healing Journey

You have likely heard a lot about acne and the commonly accepted truths about what causes it in the first place—that it's because of your skin type, hygiene, hormones, or clogged pores. We've heard, "Don't touch your face!" Or, "Don't wear makeup!" Or, "Sleep with a clean pillowcase!" We've been recommended harsh cleansers and things to zap or dry out our pimples. Not only is having so many options overwhelming, none of them seemed to work for me.

I tried implementing a lot of these suggestions. I became paranoid about ever touching my face, I washed my hands too much, I held my phone away from my face to talk, and I changed pillowcases daily. I even began consciously sleeping on my back because I heard it would help my skin breathe. I was trying everything, struggling, then trying new things, only to be left more frustrated than before.

I learned a lot, but the biggest lesson of all was that conventional wisdom about acne did not apply to my skin. In fact, a lot of the things I tried just made my skin worse. I spent a small fortune trying everything topically. I had facials almost every week and knew more about conventional acne products than I ever wanted to. Sometimes a product seemed to work for a short period of time but, inevitably, it would always stop being effective.

Before I woke up devastated by acne, I was, by all normal standards, a healthy person. I ate very well, exercised, excelled in a challenging career, and was surrounded by great friends and family. My life wasn't perfect, of course, but it certainly didn't warrant the extreme reaction that had suddenly developed on my face. After exhausting almost every topical skincare product on the market, I decided instead to make a radical change to my diet. I was desperate.

I first noticed real results by eliminating modern, chemically filled, processed foods. I saw a huge difference in just thirty days. The overall impact on my health was dramatic. Until I lived without processed foods, I didn't know how bad I felt while I had been eating them. Changing my diet changed not only my skin but also my entire perspective. I began applying the same whole, unprocessed, unpackaged, unmodified, and organic standards to everything I put on my body. I committed to healing my skin with naturally nourishing ingredients rather than with chemicals wrapped in pretty packaging.

It was a huge breakthrough.

I dug deep and learned about hidden food allergies, how modern food damages our gut health, chemical toxicity, environmental allergens, air pollutants both indoors and outdoors, skin sensitivities, and the enormous impact of stress. I came to realize how many harmful things we come into contact with every single day and that perhaps, I wasn't as healthy as I'd thought. That maybe my skin was trying to tell me something the whole time.

I now saw it was screaming at me that I needed healing from within. With acne, there is a tendency to try and scrub our faces, thinking we need to kill the acne on the surface, which exacerbates our already inflamed skin. But inflammation in the face is often caused by inflammation in the body. This insight taught me that rather than scrub my skin topically, I needed to nourish it from the inside by eating better food. Now, my rule of thumb is that if it has been changed, processed, or modified, it is not a skin-supporting food.

The last big shift in my healing happened when I started using simple techniques to manage stress and began to change my thoughts about my skin. This was the most difficult step. I shifted my attitude and adopted genuine gratitude for my skin, even though I still had acne. (Don't worry, I will teach you how to do this.) I had to practice appreciating my skin and to stop berating and attacking it. I realized that I needed to listen to it instead.

For years, I fought hard against my acne. Now I am truly grateful for the experience that allows me to help others heal their skin and become healthier in the process. I have so much more understanding and compassion than I ever did when I took my skin for granted. Reclaiming my health has been the most empowering part of the journey. However, I was only able to do that once I realized what my individual body needed to heal. I encourage you to find the same for yourself. Research everything. Investigate theories that resonate with you and trust your bodily intuition. There are endless possibilities to find healing and ultimately, happiness. Let this book guide you through your healing journey.

Let's get started!

2

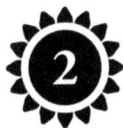

Getting Started

Don't worry too much about figuring out what "type" of acne you have, just experiment. Some things will work beautifully for you while others won't. Skin is highly individual and no one method or product works for everyone. If you've ever tried oil cleansing, you know what I'm referring to—you either love it or you hate it!

You can heal your skin from the inside out with a three-phased approach.

First, anything you put on your skin can be absorbed into your bloodstream. Products can either support your skin and overall health or challenge them both.

Second, you are what you eat. It is important that you shift your diet to one that nourishes, not ravages, your skin.

Third, your mindset and thoughts about your skin are crucial. This is the missing link for a lot of already healthy people. Though I didn't believe it at first, your thoughts have the incredible power to manifest positivity in your life. If you hate your skin, you send it a strong and stressful message. So you must repair the relationship you have with your skin and body in order to facilitate the final phases of healing.

There is no one size fits all diet or lifestyle. I discovered that I'm allergic to gluten, but it may be more beneficial for you to get rid of sugar or dairy in your diet. I'll give you a lot of options and guidance to help you find the best strategies for your skin. When people find the best foods for them, they are often pleasantly surprised when their overall health improves. While healing their skin, I have watched many people simultaneously reduce chronic pain, inflammation and seasonal allergies.

I know that acne can be a real nightmare and a major cause of stress, resulting in a loss of confidence. Once you feel like you've tried everything out there or don't know where to turn, don't lose hope. You don't need to be a scientist, nutritionist, doctor, or esthetician to create your own healing. In fact, most of my results were not through any of the training I've had. We are going to start with what you can do immediately to bring about topical relief. Then, we will work on your ideal diet and lastly, focus on your mindset. All three aspects of skincare are equally important in your skin-healing journey. Have patience, breathe, and know there is always a way—we just have to find it.

3

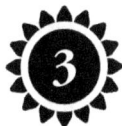

Immediate Relief

Breakouts seem to pop up at the most inopportune times. The following pages include my favorite strategies for when you need them most. I will often pick a couple of them to do up to four times a day, or whenever I have a quick moment. I have found the green tea ice cubes and essential oil spot treatment to be especially helpful for fast results.

Green Tea Ice Cubes

This is one of my favorite remedies for any type of acne. It soothes the skin, shrinks your pores, improves blood flow and reduces puffiness. It's great for under your eyes. For me, it visibly reduced inflammation and calmed my cystic acne. Green tea is high in amazing antioxidants and calming properties and ice soothes inflammation. It is also a great toner for your face and supports your skin's natural pH level.

How to Do It

1. Find an organic high-quality green tea that you love, either loose or in bags will work (follow directions on tea packaging for brewing 2 cups).

2. Heat water in a kettle to just under boiling (160-180°F) and take off of the burner.

3. You don't want the water too hot or it burns the tea and damages its properties. I just let the water boil, but then leave it on the counter for a few minutes to cool off.

4. Now, pour the water into a French press or brewing container (using only glass, ceramic, or cast iron whenever possible) and let it steep for about 10 minutes.

5. Pour the tea into ice cube molds and pop in the freezer, until frozen.

To use, wash your face and gently rub one ice cube all over your face (and neck if you'd like) until it's all melted, which only takes a few minutes. Wait until your skin warms up again before moisturizing so that it better absorbs moisture and essential oils. If I have a current breakout, I use a cube once in the morning and once in the evening for best results. If you don't have time for both, start by just trying it once a day. Enjoy your soothed face and tiny pores.

Lemon Juice and Apple Cider Vinegar

Fresh squeezed lemon juice is incredible for reducing acne scarring, red spots and cystic acne. It noticeably lightens any hyperpigmentation overnight and the juice's acidity exfoliates and regenerates the skin. It's best to try this quick-fix method at night because lemon juice can make your skin sensitive to the sun and more susceptible to burning. Because the acidity of lemon juice is strong and can damage the skin's pH balance, you'll want to use this method only periodically.

I use leftover lemon wedges from my morning lemon drink, throwing them in a glass storage container in the fridge after use. If you don't have wedges, use an organic 100% lemon juice from your fridge. (I use Santa Cruz Organic or Lakewood Organic brands.)

How to Do It

Wash your face (and use a green tea cube if you like and let your face dry), then dab the lemon wedge on the red spot you're treating. Squeeze the wedge or press it right onto your skin as a spot treatment only. If this irritates your skin, try diluting the lemon juice with water in equal portions. Avoid eyes, erupted and broken skin, and other sensitive areas.

Apple cider vinegar also works well as a spot treatment. Be sure to use only raw vinegar widely found at health food stores and even some grocery stores. (I've found Bragg Organic Apple Cider Vinegar to be best.)

Apple cider vinegar has a lot of internal health benefits as well. Most mornings, I drink warm water with 1 to 2 tablespoons of apple cider vinegar or fresh lemon juice, sometimes both. I also add a little raw organic honey. This morning drink detoxes your liver and organs and is great for supporting your digestive system. Give it a try!

KATHERINE LARSEN

Honey Mask

Raw, unfiltered, local honey is amazing. It is naturally antimicrobial, antifungal, antibacterial, and great for acne. It heals and moisturizes and is a great solution for your skin's complicated problems. While honey moisturizes dry skin, it also helps balance oily skin, all incredibly gently. Honey is amazing for healing breakouts and scarring, reducing cystic acne, and giving your skin a vibrant glow. My favorite time for a honey mask is in the bath or shower.

The best honey is local and raw because its beneficial properties are uncompromised by excessive heating and processing. Your farmers market should have good local, raw honey. A few great companies have made travel-size honey packets, like Wedderspoon and Tupelo Raw Honey Packs. I also have a tiny bear-shaped honey container from my local farmers market that I refill from my large jar of honey. Since honey is the only food on the planet that never goes bad, you can buy it in bulk. You heard me. Honey never spoils. Man, I love honey.

How to Do It

Tie back your beautiful hair, being especially careful to get all the tiny strands. Consider using a terry cloth headband too since this can get messy (though water will easily rinse the sticky honey away so don't worry too much).

Splash your face with warm water, then gently dry it with a towel until just slightly damp. Rub your hands together for about 15 seconds to warm them up. Pour about a quarter sized amount of honey into your palm, or just enough to cover your entire face, and spread gently over your face. Leave the honey on for about 20 minutes. If you're short on time, 5 to 10 minutes will still result in benefits. You can do this before you step into the shower or while you take a relaxing detox bath. Be careful not to get your face wet and the warm steam will help the honey soak in even further.

Essential Oil Spot Treatment

If you're not yet familiar with essential oils, get to know them as soon as possible. They are incredibly useful tools for cleaning, laundry, natural pest control, gardening, healing the skin, bathing, hair care, homemade soaps and home remedies. The oils I use most for skin are lavender, chamomile, and tea tree. You can get fancy with the types or buy organic, but any essential oils are better than none. Keep in mind that your skin's essential oil needs will change, especially as you support it through this healing journey.

With essential oils especially, just because it's natural doesn't always mean it's safe. Essential oils are powerful, so you don't need to use a lot. Make sure you do your research and check with your doctor before using essential oils if you are pregnant or have any health conditions.

One of my favorite books is Valerie Ann Worwood's, The Complete Book of Essential Oils and Aromatherapy. It has a ton of ideas on how to use your favorite essential oils safely. I've also found a clinical aroma therapist in my city who hosts custom blending sessions and has helped me discover one of my favorite skincare blends of lavender, ylang ylang and carrot seed oil.

Lavender essential oil is anti-inflammatory, antibacterial, antibiotic, antifungal and antiviral. It is great for facilitating healing, calming skin, and easing dry skin. These properties make it all-around amazing for acne prone skin. My favorite oil for stress relief, lavender is soothing and relaxing. I use it more than any other oil and often on my face, neck, and body.

Tea tree oil is powerful for acne treatment—especially for skin that is infected and cystic. It is also antibacterial, antibiotic, antiviral and antifungal.

Roman chamomile is another great essential oil for acne. It is best for sensitive skin, calming inflammation as it heals. It's also great at relieving stress which also helps relieve acne overall.

Other great oils for the skin are carrot seed, frankincense, neroli and, my personal favorite (the best smelling essential oil ever), ylang ylang. If you do nothing else, go get some ylang ylang and start sniffing!

I've had a lot of fun finding and perfecting new essential oil blends for my skin as well as learning about them through local stores and resources. Look around your area or Google local aroma therapists, stores and organic spas. You can even search for meetup groups in your area. I get my favorite essential oils online at Essential 3.

How to Do It

Add one or two drops of lavender oil to pure jojoba oil to moisturize your face and body. You can also put a few drops in a bath for powerful relaxation. Lavender is an amazing spot treatment for acne, scars, and broken or inflamed skin—just put one drop on the blemish and leave it alone. You can reapply lavender a few times a day.

Dab a few drops of tea tree oil directly onto a spot before bed or in the morning. If the acne is particularly bad, reapply with a drop throughout the day.

For Roman chamomile, put a drop on your skin and leave it be.

Structured Silver

Structured silver products are comprised of .0001% pure metallic silver and structured water or gel, depending on the product. Silver is highly antimicrobial and kills bacteria, viruses, yeast and some parasites. It is powerful at killing acne bacteria though extremely gentle, so it's a great solution for broken or sensitive skin. Liquid silver effectively supports your immune system when taken internally. You can also use it for internal microbial issues or add it to a soothing aloe vera gel for fast topical healing. (It's so effective that wound care companies line dressings with silver to help patients heal faster.) Make sure to read all labels and instructions.

How to Do It

1. If using the gel form, smooth the silver gel on your face at night after washing it or in the morning wherever you have a breakout. (It will feel heavy if you use too much so I like to use it at night.)

2. If you have the liquid form, you can pour it into a glass spray bottle (not plastic) and spritz your face, focusing on your troubled areas. I love adding 1-2 drops of tea tree essential oil per 1-2 ounces of water for extra antibacterial power.

Stretchy Cotton Mask

A cotton mask is wonderful for infusing moisture and essential oils deep into your skin while minimizing acne and blackheads. (You'll need a special kind of stretchy cotton that I was able to find on Amazon called Selena Multi-layer Cotton Puffs.) Using this mask frequently has dramatically improved my complexion. It also seems to diminish congestion and improve the appearance of blackheads. It's great for when you have a big evening event, you are feeling very dry or your skin needs some extra love.

How to Do It

1. Grab about 5 layers of the stretchy cotton squares.

2. Pour about 1/8th cup of filtered water into a small glass dish.

3. Add 1-2 drops of the essential oil of your choice. (I like lavender and chamomile.)

4. Dip the cotton squares into the water until they're fully soaked and gently press out the excess water.

5. Place about a quarter sized amount of facial moisturizer on the squares.

6. Peel apart the layers of the squares about halfway, then smooth the two halves together like a sandwich. Then pull apart the next layer and repeat. The idea here is that you want to get some lotion on each of the five squares.

7. Now, one by one, carefully stretch out a square, then apply it to your face in the following order: cheeks, forehead, across the nose, and then over your nose and chin, with a small hole for your mouth.

8. Rub your hands together for about 15 seconds until warm and place them on your cheeks for 15-30 seconds so that the heat infuses the essential oils and lotion into your skin. You can even make a "ha" sound, cupping your hands together for a little extra heat. Unleash your inner Darth Vader.

9. Leave the mask on for exactly 3 minutes, no more. If any lotion remains on your face, gently smooth it into your skin.

Gelatin Mask

Gelatin is an animal protein rich in collagen that's found in the connective tissues. It heals in many ways and can be used for gelatin masks.

Modern diets lack this once widely used source of protein. I add gelatin to my diet by melting it in tea, coffee, warm soups or smoothies. It has made a big difference in my overall health and skin. I highly recommend taking a few tablespoons daily.

How to Do It

1. Pour 1 tablespoon of warm filtered water and ½ a tablespoon of lemon juice in a small glass bowl.

2. Immediately mix in ½ a tablespoon of gelatin and stir until dissolved.

3. If any gelatin clumps remain, remove them before applying and throw into the garbage, not the sink or it could clog.

4. Smooth the gelatin mask onto your clean face and leave on for 20 minutes. Rinse with warm water, then marvel at your youthful skin!

Clay Mask

Clay is an ancient detoxifier and beauty secret. Clay is especially helpful for blackheads and congested pores. Types include green clay for oilier skin, pink kaolin clay for dry or sensitive skin, and bentonite clay for normal to oily skin. For extra healing power, there's a great high-end clay mask called Alitura. Try a few to find one that works best for you.

Using a clay mask once a week is a great way to pull toxins out of your skin. I can often see an immediate difference in how clear my skin looks. You can also use it as a very small spot treatment overnight. Throw a towel over your pillowcase or just use an old one, as the clay can rub off. I don't recommend doing this mask in the shower or bath because the extra moisture can prevent the clay from drying.

How to Do It

In a small glass or wooden bowl, mix 1-2 tablespoons of bentonite clay with 2 teaspoons of water, or enough to make a medium-thick paste. Do not use metal bowls or spoons as they can weaken the effects of the clay. For extra healing and calming properties, add a few drops of lavender, tea tree or any other essential oil with which you've had success. You can use apple cider vinegar in place of, or along with, the water, but be careful if your skin tends to be sensitive or dry. Cover your face and as much of your neck as you'd like and leave on for 20 minutes or until dry. You will feel your face tighten and pulse as it dries. This is normal and means the clay is powerfully at work. After 20 minutes, gently splash your face with warm water until the clay softens enough to wash away.

Your skin may be red for about 30-60 minutes after this treatment. If your skin feels too dry, use some jojoba oil before bed to restore moisture.

Facial Steam

Dealing with acne, you are often left with scabbing or scarring. When trying to get your skin to its best before a big event and plagued with the aftermath of your last breakout, soften up some of the damage with a facial steam.

A facial steam is an easy and inexpensive at-home spa treatment by boiling water in a saucepan or tea kettle. The warmth of the steam opens up your pores, allowing your skin to drink in moisture, essential oils, or whatever nourishing treatment you are trying. As a bonus, I've found that adding tea tree oil to the water is effective for battling respiratory illness. Inhaling the tea tree helps kill the funk when you're just not feeling well.

How to Do It

Fill a medium saucepan halfway full with filtered water until boiling, then turn off the heat. Be careful not to burn yourself. Feel with your hand to gauge the ideal distance you should sit from the pan for steam that's warm and relaxing, not hot or scalding. Add any essential oils, using just a few drops per batch. With a towel, create a little healing tent to trap and direct the steam toward your face. Steam for about 10 minutes. After, take advantage of your open pores by applying your favorite serum or moisturizer, mixing in a drop of essential oil if you wish. Apply green tea ice cubes to seal in the good stuff and close up your pores.

If you're short on time, add extra water to your tea kettle when making your morning drink. Once the kettle has begun to steam, use your hand to find a safe distance and then slowly and very cautiously place your face into the steam coming from the kettle while it's singing. Start with your face high and gently lower it to find where the steam is just warm enough. Hold it there for

1-2 minutes, then immediately apply essential oils, moisturizer, or whatever you're using for the day. If your skin is struggling, you can do a green tea ice cube treatment after your steam to calm it down and reduce inflammation.

Estheticians and Spas

When you're in a pinch and your skin is driving you crazy, the right esthetician can be very helpful. Find an esthetician who can perform a gentle facial or extractions and be very picky. Call natural or holistic spas and ask about the products they use, then research the brands and ingredients online. You may have to fight their suggestions for chemical peels, microdermabrasions, or other harsh methods. Trust me, it's not worth it—you'll get the best results with the gentlest methods.

Estheticians are mainly trained to use conventional products which are full of chemicals. Even many high-end organic and natural products negatively affected my skin. When I explained to my esthetician that I regained my health by cutting out chemicals and modified ingredients, she understood and it greatly improved my experience. You're paying for a service—advocate for your preferences, or spend your money elsewhere.

....

A Note on Picking

Even though we know we shouldn't, we've all done it. I'm talking about picking, or performing home surgery on your blemishes. The struggle is real, but you will be much better off if you can talk yourself out of it. Picking only makes the skin more inflamed, causing scabbing and scarring and increasing your skin's recovery time. When you have the urge, tell yourself that you can try home extractions if you'd like but first, try doing something to reduce your stress about the breakout. Go outside for a walk, drink some tea, do a breathing technique, or take a long bath. Then weigh the benefits and hopefully you'll decide to give your skin another day to heal before intervening.

For the occasional home extraction, gently but thoroughly wash your face and hands first. To keep from directly touching your exposed skin, use tissue between your index fingers, which helps your grip and prevents infection. Remember, any opening in your skin is a chance for infection and inflammation. Do not pick or scrape at the top layer of your skin. Instead, gently push down at the base of either side of the blemish. Try only three times. If nothing clears, it is not ready and you will only inflame the blemish more. Relax and try again tomorrow.

Attempting extractions yourself will cause inflammation and visible redness, so do this at night when your pores are at their fullest and have many hours to calm and relax. Follow with direct pressure on the blemish for about thirty seconds to minimize swelling or bleeding, then place an ice cube on the spot you just extracted to reduce inflammation (green tea cubes are best). Finally, put a drop of lavender essential oil on the area and let it rest.

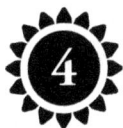

Skincare Routines

The healthy things you do in your life each day add up over time for a big difference. The same holds true for your skin. Treating it well every day with simple, gentle products and consistent care will help your skin heal dramatically.

First, in the spirit of loving your skin, let's talk about eyes and makeup removal. The skin around your eyes is incredibly delicate and thin so you want to be gentle in that area to keep your skin healthy and youthful.

If you're wearing eye makeup, first apply a small amount of coconut oil to the makeup around your eyelashes and lids to coat. Then use a soft tissue to wipe up the black mess. Keep applying and gently wipe away the makeup until your eyes are clean and clear. Then, wash away the oil with water and gentle castile soap (see my favorite brand in the Resource Guide), just around your eyes. You can also use a microfiber mitt to gently clear your pores of any residual makeup. However, I don't like to use the microfiber mitt very much for dark eye makeup because it can stain your mitt, but foundation and concealer don't typically stain.

To perfect this skincare routine, it took many years of trying something new, breaking out, adjusting and then moving on to the next method—from oil cleansing, only gentle soaps, hypoallergenic lines, herbs, paleo skincare lines, organic products, gluten-free, you name it. I have found the following methods to be the best, hands down.

Washing Your Face

1. Pull back your hair and splash your face with warm water. With wet hands, pour about a quarter sized amount of organic raw honey into your palms (or enough to cover your face), and then gently rub it all over your face, just as you would with soap. Rinse off the honey with lukewarm water, being careful around your eyes as it can sometimes sting.

2. To help with inflammation, puffy eyes and breakouts, apply a green tea ice cube all over your face until it melts. Wait until your skin is warm before proceeding.

3. Pour a small amount of jojoba oil, smaller than the size of a nickel, into your palms and rub them together briskly to warm the oil. You can mix the jojoba oil with a drop of lavender or another essential oil blend. Then apply it to your face.

Don't be concerned about applying base or carrier oils to your face. The key is finding the right type of oil. For myself and many others, jojoba oil has been the best overall. It doesn't make me breakout or congested. Though pricey, healing argan oil can be used in small amounts (a little goes a long way). A minimal amount of castor oil or rosehip seed oil can be beneficial as well. Just blend a small amount of any of these oils, about 5-15%, into jojoba oil and experiment. Oils that caused skin congestion for me were olive, neem, tamanu and, even my favorite for many things, coconut. However, oils that work best for you will be highly individual.

No Soap Microfiber Face Mitt Method

Every day, after using the honey method above, I use a gentle microfiber hand mitt that has made a big difference in my routine. (I use a Jane Iredale Magic Mitt that can be found on Amazon.) Great for sensitive skin, a microfiber mitt clears any residual makeup not removed with the honey washing method, deeply cleans pores, helps with blackheads and gently exfoliates your skin. And since you aren't using soap, the natural acid mantle of your skin isn't disrupted. It also feels like a luxurious treat for your skin. Some clients have had great success by using the microfiber face mitt as the only way they clean their face and don't ever use face wash, toners or moisturizers. Simple and cost effective!

How to Do It

First, make sure you've removed any eye makeup with either coconut oil or gentle castile soap. Rinse your mitt with warm water only, then slowly and gently rub it on your skin in circular motions to remove any face makeup (foundation, concealer, powder), being extra gentle on the sensitive area around your eyes. Pay attention as to whether you can see foundation, concealer or powder makeup darkening your mitt as your skin becomes super clean. Continue until you no longer see transferred makeup. Be sure to immediately clean your mitt with a mild castile soap like Dr. Bronner's and then hang it to dry before your next use.

Oil Cleansing

Oil cleansing is an ancient form of face washing that may sound crazy initially. The idea is that like dissolves like, so by putting oil on your face, you're helping to dissolve the oil on your skin. I did oil cleansing when my skin was still pretty bad with acne and it helped a lot. The key is finding the right oils for your skin and using very warm (but comfortable) water.

For basic oil cleansing, you'll need a clean washcloth and a carrier oil, like jojoba. Deciding which oil to use is an individual thing. For acne prone skin, I recommend first trying jojoba oil, rosehip seed oil or argan oil. Do not use processed or heated industrial seed oils like canola, corn, soy or cottonseed. You can use a small amount of argan oil mixed in with jojoba oil for extra moisturizing and healing (try 90% jojoba to 10% argan). Castor oil is great to add to jojoba oil in a ratio of 80% jojoba oil to 20% castor oil. Tamanu oil was also great for me as a healing spot treatment, but not for my entire face since it seemed to make my skin congested. You can try and see how one oil works for you before blending. I recommend starting with a high quality jojoba oil.

A good basic rule of thumb for cleansing oils is if it's not considered a "paleo diet" approved oil, I would not recommend trying it on your skin. I've also found that certain oils can be better or worse for acne prone skin, depending on the oleic acid to linoleic acid ratio of the oil. Some people with acne do better with oils higher in linoleic acid. If jojoba doesn't work for you after a few weeks, try experimenting with other oils. Oil cleansing is very much an individual process.

I use oil cleansing intermittently as a way to beat dry winter skin or refresh skin that's looking a little tired or worn out. I love oil cleansing in the shower where I don't have to worry about getting oil on anything, especially my hair. If you have very short or thin hair, proceed with caution—the oil can give your hair an overall greasy look. Try this one on a weekend or a day off when you have some time. There can be an adjustment period with any new skin routine so try it for about a week before determining if it works for you.

How to Do It

First, make sure any eye makeup is removed using the method described in the beginning of this chapter. Pour about a nickel sized amount of oil (or enough to cover your face) into your clean hands and rub them together briefly, just enough to warm the oil. Now, apply the oil to your entire face. Massage the oil into your face with gentle, upward, circular strokes for a minute or two. If you have time, now is a great time to multi-task with a short lymph massage (explained later in this chapter).

Next, run your washcloth under very warm water (but not uncomfortably hot) and ring it out. Hold the washcloth over your face for about thirty seconds, or up to two minutes, and then start to gently wipe away the oil from your face. You'll want to rinse as much oil as you can from the cloth with warm water again and continue to wipe the oil away from your face until it feels clear. It's fine to leave a little oil on your face depending on how your skin feels. If your skin doesn't feel moisturized enough, add a few small drops of oil to your face to moisturize. Always make sure to wash your washcloth thoroughly with a gentle castile soap between each use. I recommend machine washing your washcloth every week.

Simple Soap Method

If you really like using soap, or any product that lathers, you'll need to pay special attention to its effect on your skin. The lathering agents can strip your skin of its natural oils and protective barrier, which disrupts your skin's pH balance, resulting in breakouts. Follow the steps below to try my favorite gentle castile soap and how to restore the natural pH of your skin after cleansing.

How to Do It

1. Dilute a gentle soap like Dr. Bronner's Almond Castile Soap. Avoid using Dr. Bronner's citrus or peppermint versions on your face since they include real essential oils and can burn your eyes. Make a solution of 1 part soap and 4 parts water. I've also enjoyed using Miracle II Moisturizing Soap (listed in the Resource Guide), which does not need to be diluted.

2. Rub a green tea ice cube on your face and neck until it melts. Wait a few minutes for the green tea to soak into your skin and your skin to warm back up. Or, try another method listed in the next section for a balance restoring toner.

3. If using a moisturizer, jojoba oil is my favorite. Rub your hands together vigorously for 20-30 seconds to warm them. Pour about a nickel sized or less amount of jojoba, or your favorite oil from the oil cleansing method section, into your hands. You can also use a light, clean lotion like M2 Miracle Lotion (listed in the Resource Guide). Then, add a drop or two of lavender oil, tea tree oil, or your favorite essential oil blend. Rub the mixture together before gently applying it to your face. I hold my palms over my cheeks and my fingers over my forehead for 20-30 seconds to let the heat from my hands help the moisture sink in, sometimes cupping my hands and using the heat of my breath.

4. If your skin is extra challenged or dry, consider using the Stretchy Cotton Mask treatment in chapter 3 in place of step 3.

Toners

If you use a toner, here are a few options to try between cleansing and moisturizing. Apple cider vinegar helps balance the skin's pH and can naturally battle bacteria, infection, and other unwanted bad guys camping out on your face. Be sure to use an organic, raw apple cider vinegar (like Bragg's) found in health food stores. Dilute the vinegar with the same amount of filtered water, then saturate a cotton ball or tissue and gently swipe across your face, keeping far away from your eyes. If you have broken skin or sensitive areas, this will seriously sting so proceed cautiously.

Witch hazel is another favorite toner. It is antimicrobial, has natural astringent properties, and helps tighten your face and pores. Make sure you read the ingredients on the witch hazel you buy— some are combined with extra ingredients and other stuff that diminish the quality. See the Resource Guide for my favorite one.

Making Your Routine Sacred

Stay with me on this. I've found that when I'm calm, present, and breathing deeply through the steps of my skincare routine, my skin responds even better.

We'll talk about the effect of stress on your skin later but, for now, breathe deeply and relax while going through your routine. This prep time is sometimes the only moment in the day you have to yourself, so make it peaceful.

Your bathroom space is important, a place in which you spend a lot of time over the course of your life. Find ways to make it special, comfortable and visually pleasing. It will have a positive psychological effect that sends a message to your body that your skin is valued and cherished.

The goal is to pamper your skin with simple, little things. It doesn't have to be expensive. Just make any upgrades to your space that you can. Here are some of my favorite ways to upgrade a bathroom.

- Buy beautiful, decorative glass bottles for your liquid soap or shampoo. Use decorative jars or small, pretty containers.

- Hang fresh or dried herbs on your shower head with a ribbon or rubber band. Use lavender for relaxation and stress relief or eucalyptus for an invigorating and deep-breathing experience. Look around Pinterest or Google for ideas, but have fun. It can be decorative or functional or both.

- Check out the lighting in your bathroom. Soft, warm lighting makes your skin look better, and you'll feel better about it. Replace fluorescent lighting with soft incandescent light, or encourage natural sunlight. Invest in different lighting options. If you live in an apartment, buy a small lamp.

- Make sure you like your towels. Buy a special towel for your face. Keep it clean and change it often. Pick colors that make you feel happy or calm, whatever you need most.

- Hang a picture of something you love. Surround yourself with positive messages, uplifting images, and beautiful colors. Paint your walls a calming or uplifting color with nontoxic paint.

- Keep your space clean and organized. Clutter raises your stress levels. Make sure your bathtub is clean for relaxing baths. Hire a cleaning service to help you clean or find a fun way to get partners, children, or friends engaged in this project together. Sometimes the hardest part is asking for help and being alright with not trying to do it all yourself.

- Get an indoor plant for your bathroom. Plants upgrade your space and purify indoor air.

- Buy beautiful, handcrafted soaps. Indulge your senses and make your routine an experience. I love finding local handcrafted soaps at my farmer's market. Whole Foods, and other health food stores, carry many natural soaps that are rich in color and scents. One of my favorites is Zum Bar Goat's Milk Coffee-Almond Soap.

- Buy candles for natural lighting next to your sink or on the ledge of the bathtub. Go for natural, organic scents made from essential oils (think recognizable herbs and spices). Skip paraffin candles as they can emit toxic fumes. Opt instead for natural beeswax candles—ancient air purifiers that emit negative ions. I find locally sourced beeswax candles at my farmer's market or local health food store. If you're into do-it-yourself projects, making your own beeswax candles is pretty simple. Make sure the beeswax is ethically and safely sourced. (Google "Colony Collapse Disorder" for the full story on why bees are at risk of becoming extinct.)

Weekly Routines

Detox Bath

A soothing, relaxing detox bath is one of my favorite skincare and overall health rituals. It pulls toxins out of your body, softens your skin and exfoliates dead skin cells. It's great for overworked muscles, generalized pain, water retention or if you're feeling a cold or flu coming on. After a detox bath I feel much lighter, so relaxed and I sleep like a baby.

How to Do It

Fill your clean bathtub full of very warm water. You don't want it to be scalding but you're going to be in there for 20-30 minutes so it will cool down a bit. While the tub is filling, add about 1 cup of Epsom salts or Dead Sea salts. (I use unscented Dr. Teals. If you want a scent, add a few drops of essential oils.)

If desired, add about 2 teaspoons of a liquid trace mineral supplement called ConcenTrace Trace Mineral Drops, which is a great way to absorb 72 different trace minerals while enjoying your bath. If taking a bath at night, consider adding about 2 tablespoons of magnesium chloride salts or magnesium flakes. (I use Health & Wisdom Magnesium Bath Crystals.) But be careful: you may get very sleepy at first.

Next, pour in a liquid soap like Dr. Bronner's or Miracle II Moisturizing Soap, aiming it at the stream from the running bath to get maximum bubbles. You'll love the feeling of sinking into a bath full of sudsy goodness. While the bath is filling, do some dry body brushing. (See Dry Body Brushing in Chapter 7.)

After turning off the water, pour in about 1 cup of baking soda to both neutralize any chemicals in the water and soften your skin. Then, add about five drops of an essential oil like lavender or Roman chamomile for its relaxing, healing qualities. Both are great for helping you decompress after a long day. Wait 3-5 minutes, then step in. Set a timer for 20-30 minutes (at the most) so you don't have to worry about staying in too long or falling asleep. Close your eyes and breathe deeply. Remember, this is your time to relax—nowhere to go, nothing else to do. Clear your mind and soak up this experience. Know you are doing something excellent for your body and mind.

Relaxing in the tub is an excellent time for a honey face mask or a moisturizing hair treatment since you'll be there for at least 20 minutes and won't have to worry about anything dripping on the floor. Have fun finding new ways to treat yourself.

A wonderful way to end your bath is with a powerful body exfoliation treatment which will further aid your body in detoxing. When your timer rings and while your tub is draining, use an exfoliating mitt to scrub away any softened, dead skin. I found an incredible exfoliator on Amazon called Asian Magic Exfoliating Bath and Shower Washcloths. They last a long time and are very effective. They work best on slightly damp skin. You can use a small amount of soap on the cloth while either scrubbing or after you're all done exfoliating. You just want to make sure you wash all the toxins off your body after the detox bath. You may find the exfoliating process somewhat gross the first time you do it, but remember: the dead skin and other gunk is always better out than in!

Start with your feet and work your way up toward your heart using both small circular motions and long upward strokes. When your cloth has collected too much dead skin, just rinse it off and keep going until you don't see any more dead skin on the cloth. Then, move to a new patch of skin and repeat. When you get to your stomach, use clockwise circular motions. To scrub your arms, start with your fingers and move up your arm. Be very gentle on your underarms. If you've just shaved, then skip that area. Stop close to your neckline, avoiding your face. Always avoid any sensitive areas.

Exfoliating can be harsh on your skin so I don't advise doing it more than once per week. You should also limit your detox baths to weekly. Make sure you hydrate with pure filtered water after your bath and step out of the tub slowly and carefully. If you feel dizzy or weak after your bath, the water was probably too hot or you stayed in the bath too long. Reduce the temperature next time and make sure you do a lot of rehydrating if you don't feel well.

After your bath, treat your skin to food grade organic virgin coconut oil, shea butter or jojoba oil as a moisturizer (or any other clean chemical-free, high quality lotion). You can put a drop of essential oil into your palm and mix it with your moisturizer or lotion for an even better at home spa experience. Your skin especially needs to rehydrate and drink in moisture after your detox bath. Now, marvel at your soft, youthful, smooth skin!

....

A Note on Detox Baths

It's been said that the best practice is to shower first before you get into a detox bath. The idea is that showering removes dirt and oil from your skin so that you're not soaking in it. I have found this to be impractical if you have only one shower or bath, or just too time consuming. After an especially sweaty workout, I may take a quick shower first, but you'll still feel the benefits of a detox bath by forgoing a shower beforehand.

Also, it's a great investment is to use a water filter for your shower or bath. I use a Structured Water Filter (see the Resource Guide) which differs greatly from conventional filters in many ways and does not require a replacement filter. I don't have a filter on my bathtub faucet, just on the showerhead. I fill my tub partially with the structured/filtered water from the shower head to help with the unfiltered water from the tub. (A small amount of structured water can positively affect unstructured water when combined.) If you don't have filtered water in your bathroom, adding the baking soda previously mentioned helps neutralize chemicals like chlorine. If you can afford it, I highly recommend investing in a whole-house structured water system or at least a basic filter. We absorb the chemicals in our tap water and if you're having skin or hair issues, your water may be the cause.

. . . .

Facial Exfoliation Options

If your face feels dry or dull or appears lackluster, exfoliate the dead skin cells weekly to give the fresh new skin underneath a chance to shine. Weekly exfoliation helps open clogged pores, blackheads and whiteheads. Baking soda is an effective and inexpensive exfoliator. (I use Bob's Red Mill or sometimes Arm & Hammer.) Wash your face, leaving it damp, then pour a nickel sized amount of baking soda into your palm. Gently—and I mean gently—rub the baking soda on your face in a circular, upward motion. After about thirty seconds, rinse with lukewarm water and follow with a moisturizer. Be careful if you're using essential oils in your skincare regimen because your skin will be very sensitive after exfoliating. If your face feels sore, make sure to be more gentle next time and try blending the baking soda with jojoba oil instead of water. Use a green tea ice cube for a toner afterward if your skin feels sensitive. Otherwise, you can use apple cider vinegar or witch hazel for a toner. Toning after the baking soda exfoliation is key to balancing your skin's pH.

If your acne is inflamed or your skin broken, you'll want to proceed with caution. Know that it's best to calm down your skin, not further agitate it. Never use a body scrub for your face—the granules are too big and harsh and can damage your skin and make acne worse. Even if it's a homemade sea salt or sugar scrub, it's still not meant for your face.

Once-In-A-While Routines

A major contributor to my acne was the overall toxic load of chemicals on my body. I found that the more I worked to reduce my toxin and chemical exposure, the better my skin responded. Everything you encounter through food, skin care and your environment has to be processed through your body's detox pathways. So, if your liver, kidneys and gut are not able to handle all the toxins, the skin steps in to help.

A great intermittent detox strategy is using a far infrared sauna. You can find one at a local spa. If you love it, you can purchase one online for your home. Far infrared differs from other saunas in its ability to raise your body temperature from the inside out, instead of heating your body from the outside in. The powerful far infrared heat helps your body detox and sweat, supports your health, and increases circulation. It boosts the lymphatic system and improves your skin tone. These saunas should not be used if you have any major health issues, heart or lung conditions, are pregnant or think you might be. Always check with your physician first before trying any kind of sauna or hot/cold treatment described in this section.

Make sure to hydrate before and after using a far infrared sauna, and use only with the proper instruction of a professional. If you decide to buy your own, make sure you read your manual and follow instructions. These saunas can be dangerous if not used properly.

They can also be incredibly drying and damaging to your hair. To prevent hair issues, wet your hair, put in a deep conditioning treatment, and wrap it all up in a wet towel before entering the sauna. When you're done, shower to wash away all the toxins you've released onto your skin through sweating and rinse the conditioning treatment from your hair.

Steam saunas can also have a great effect on your skin. This is especially true if your skin is sensitive or dry. Wash your face, put on a very light moisturizer, and then go into the steam room for 10-20 minutes. Steam saunas are great for sweating out toxins and getting moisture at the same time. Again, be careful and proceed with caution.

Massage is another intermittent treat to add to your routine. Relaxing treatments are great in general because they help enable your body's innate healing capabilities. Massage helps boost your circulation, improves lymphatic drainage, reduces stress and decreases cortisol levels. Lowering both your stress and cortisol has a positive effect on reducing acne.

Hot-Cold Detox Plunges

I know this won't be a routine option for most of us, but hot and cold plunges are great if you're on vacation. I experienced them first in Costa Rica. I had stepped on a sea urchin and my foot was full of poisonous barbs. (Best. Vacation. Ever.) After limping around, I went to the natural hot springs at the base of a mountain. Our guide explained the ancient detoxification properties of quickly going from the hot to cold pools. We spent the entire afternoon there because it felt so good. If you have access to hot tubs or steam rooms and a cold pool or lake, simply quickly go from one to the other, hot to cold. However, to avoid absorbing chemicals, don't do this with a community pool that uses chlorine or other chemicals.

This is not for the faint of heart! I've included plunges and showers because they are free, are fast, and have worked wonders for me.

Cold Thermogenesis

Some crazy people out there take ice baths to get the benefits of the theory of cold thermogenesis. It's only crazy if it doesn't work though, right? Well, the results can be amazing and the big impact for most is weight loss. However, cold also helps reduce inflammation and improves the quality of your skin. What I've noticed with using cold strategies is improved circulation and skin tone, less dryness, more energy, increased mood and better thought clarity. It will also wake you up in a flash if you're short on sleep!

How to Do It

To get the benefits by taking a cold shower, turn the water down gradually, just enough to feel a moderate difference. Make 3-5 temperature adjustments in about a minute. Once the water is icy cold, back into the shower stream so that your shoulders are the first thing to hit the cold water. The shoulders and back of the neck are key spots in getting your body's temperature to drop. Gradually back in to the point where your whole body is under the cold shower entirely. Stand in the shower for 3 minutes. You can work up to it.

Dave Aspery of the Bulletproof Executive offers another way to get the same overall anti-inflammatory benefits of cold thermogenesis. Fill up a container full of cold water and dump ice cubes or chips into the water. Hold your face in the water for as long as you can stand it or hold your breath. This is highly effective for extra care, but so very cold! (Google Bulletproof Executive Ice Face to read more.)

Lymph Massages

Your body's lymph system naturally detoxes and carries waste out of your system. It is unique in that it requires movement in order to move the toxins out of your body. Exercise is one great way to move your lymph; so is rebounding, which is very fun and involves jumping on a trampoline. I have found lymph massage to help with clearing blockages and acne.

Once you learn where the lymph points are located, pay attention to whether yours feel blocked, swollen, achy, or full. I can tell when I've overindulged or haven't consumed enough water because the area under my chin by my ears becomes swollen, feeling "stuck." It's important to always massage these points gently.

How to Do It

1. Start under the point of your chin with both thumbs pressing up and your palms together, as if praying. Pressing up gently right inside your jaw bone, move both thumbs along the inside of your jaw until you get to your ears on each side. You can lightly feel the lymph nodes, especially if they are swollen and tender.

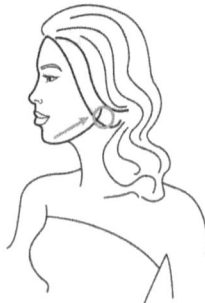

2. When you get to your ears, press on the hollow spaces directly below each ear, releasing the lymph from this area.

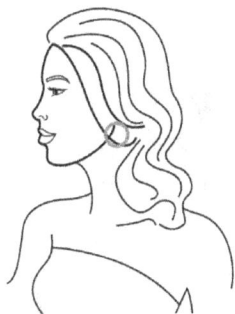

3. Then, with your opposite hand, making sure your finger tips are flat and together, press down from the bottoms of your ears along your neck, all the way to the tops of your shoulders, as if massaging your neck. Do this on both sides.

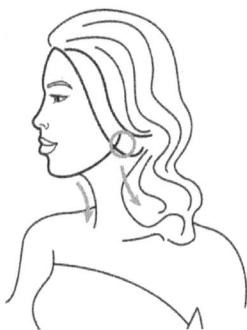

4.   Starting at the center of your collarbone, right under the "u" shape in the middle, run your fingers vertically right below the top ridge, moving outward. Do this on both sides.

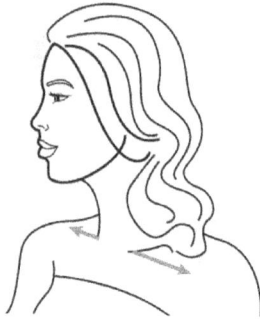

5.   Next, gently pinch the fronts of your armpits, in the crease shown in the figure, to drain the lymph. Once complete, you can start over with step 1 and go through the steps a few times. Then, make sure to drink a glass of pure water to help your body flush the toxins. The whole process is quick enough to do whenever you think about it, or when your face feels sluggish and dull.

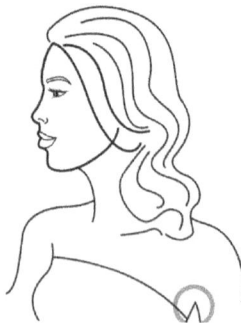

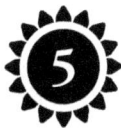

5

Clean Makeup

The goal of this book is to prevent your breakouts and to heal your skin so that you don't need any makeup, right? Right! However, every journey takes time so let's learn about some options for when you want to cover up.

Here is my approach to makeup: I don't wear any on the days I stay home, letting my skin breathe as much as possible which helps a lot. If I'm going out, I may put on a few dabs of spot concealer, if needed, and some blush or mascara—that's about it. Days where I have a meeting or an event, I will use spot concealer, mineral powder, mascara, sometimes eyeliner, and glossy lipstick. I recommend you start to simplify your makeup as much as you're comfortable with.

I used to buy high-end department counter makeup full of beautifully bright colors which performed well, so I know how good makeup should look and feel. In my quest for going natural, I've tried and learned a lot. While clean, quality ingredients are most important, you don't have to sacrifice what the makeup is supposed to do in the first place: help you look your best. One of the biggest things I appreciate about making the switch to natural products is that instead of judging a product by its bad ingredients, you get to see how many skin supporting, good ingredients there are. For example, I use products that are made of skin superfoods like argan oil, shea butter, cocoa butter, or essential oils.

The Environmental Working Group's online Skin Deep Cosmetics Database is a great resource for learning about makeup and body products. EWG rates skin products based on toxicity and the potential danger of its ingredients. Search for a specific product or ingredient to see an overall rating.

Could your makeup actually make you healthier? Maybe! Here are the clean products that I recommend.

100% Pure

This is my favorite all-around makeup brand. The company uses fruit pigments for color and they turn out vibrant and beautiful. Some of its mascaras contain gluten so be careful if you have an allergy.

The lip glazes are amazing! My go-to colors are Cherry (which I'm wearing on the back cover of this book), Raspberry, and Cabernet. These moisturizing lipsticks have just the right amount of gloss and shine. I often put on a clean lip balm first so that the color is not quite as bright for daily wear. I buy mine from the 100% Pure website or Amazon.

RMS Beauty

This is one of the cleanest foundation brands I've found. The coverage is great. The key to making any makeup work for you is finding the right color to match your skin's natural tone and for my fair skin and warm undertone, I use the "Un" Cover-Up, a tiny container of cream foundation, in Shade 11 for winter to Shade 22 for summer. Simply dab this concealer/foundation on troubled spots or discolorations before brushing on a mineral powder over your entire face. Another RMS product I love is called Lip2Cheek which is a combination lip color and cream blush. I like the color Smile. This cream blush stays on better than powder and is great for dry skin.

Caren Minerals Pure Earth Mineral Makeup

I use this powder foundation in light for winter and in medium for summer. I also use the Spice mineral blush. I highly recommend using its natural mineral makeup brushes for a smoother, more consistent coverage. While popular, mineral makeups are not created equal. This mineral foundation is made with much cleaner ingredients than the popular mineral makeup brands found in the big stores.

Eye Makeup

My favorite mascara is ZuZu Luxe which lengthens, thickens, and defines and is widely available at Whole Foods. I also like Afterglow Pure Soul in Mink and I apply a few coats for maximum effect. This one is better for darkening and defining, but not for thickening or lengthening. If you're not sensitive to gluten, 100% Pure makes a black tea mascara that thickens and lengthens really well but is more prone to smudging. After applying mascara, I run an eyelash comb through my lashes to help with clumping (since I'm still searching for the perfect natural mascara). When I'm using eyeliner, I like 100% Pure Creamstick in Pewter or any of the 100% Pure eyeliner colors.

Knowing Your Skin Type

I know this sounds basic but once I figured out that my skin needed a lot more moisture, it really started to glow. For oily skin, use powders and matte finishes. If your skin is dry, opt for cream and liquid foundations. When you're having a bad breakout, hydrate and use cream concealer, then gently brush on foundation powder. This creates a great overall coverage and will help you feel positive and confident for the day.

If you need help with your makeup, visit a natural salon or spa and have a professional do your makeup once. Ask questions to figure out your ideal colors and skin tone. It's definitely worth it one time to figure out the best techniques for you and colors that work well with your eyes, hair and skin tone.

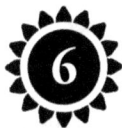

The Food Connection

When it comes to acne, if your gut is off, your skin will be too. My approach is twofold. First, we need to determine whether you have hidden food triggers or any digestive challenges. Second, after removing those damaging foods, we need to repair your gut by adding healing foods.

Modern food is drastically different from what our ancestors ate, and it's been changed in such a short period of time that our bodies haven't yet adapted to these processed foods. Allergens and foods that commonly trigger dysbiosis include grains, dairy, sugar, alcohol, soy, and genetically modified (GMO) and pesticide-laden food. Start by immediately paying attention to how the food you're eating is making you feel. Then, consider conducting an elimination diet. It is one of the best things you can do for your overall health and was a huge turning point for me. As soon as possible, test yourself for food allergies by eliminating different types of foods for a minimum of twenty-one days. After, add them back in one at a time. It is important to know that blood testing for food allergies can be inaccurate and that many people receive false negatives. By conducting your own testing through an elimination diet, you can feel what your body positively responds to and what it doesn't. Being your own detective gives you the clearest answers on how foods truly affect your body. Not only is it amazing what you can learn about yourself by conducting an elimination diet but the process is crucial for lifelong health.

....

People often ask whether they have to remove all of the common allergen foods at once or if they can just remove one. Say, go dairy free for twenty-one days but still eat gluten, sugar, and soy. For many reasons, this approach does not work. You need to clean up the entire environment of your body to see the impact of certain foods when adding them back in. For example, think of a child's very messy bedroom. If you throw one piece of trash onto the floor amidst the clutter and chaos, you don't really notice that one piece. However, imagine the room is clean and pristine. Now, throw one piece of trash onto the floor and it's all you can see. The impact is this dramatic when doing an elimination diet.

....

It's best to start with gluten and grains, dairy, sugar, alcohol, soy, peanuts, and legumes. Don't worry—it's not as hard as it sounds, and your body is more than worth it. For support, ideas, and what to expect, I recommend the Whole30 Program (paleo diet), the Clean program (alkaline diet), or the Immune System Recovery Plan (autoimmune supporting diet).

When my skin had its first huge breakout, I had been vegetarian for about six years, ate whole grains, drank soy milk, bought cage-free eggs, ate mostly organic and loved salads. I rarely ate fast food or dessert. I worked out five or six days a week doing yoga, CrossFit, and P90X. I frequented my local health food store and saw my chiropractor weekly. So, I thought I should have been feeling pretty good. However, I experienced severe digestive pain, extreme fatigue, brain fog, crippling chronic pain, and tons of seasonal allergies among many other issues. Then, the development of my acne overnight was the final straw. I tried so many products and expensive spa facials but nothing seemed to work consistently. My friends and family tried not to say anything, but sometimes even they couldn't help it.

Desperate and a real mess, I jumped on the opportunity when my CrossFit friends did a thirty day whole food challenge. I struggled knowing that I would have to ditch being vegetarian but my desperation and nagging intuition that something inside of me was really off were the deciding factors. I first tried baked chicken and realized that it was one of the only things that didn't make my stomach hurt. I had nothing to lose at this point. I had researched the amazing stories of lives being changed forever on an elimination diet of whole, ancient, Paleolithic foods and I wanted that for myself. So I eliminated all grains, dairy, soy, legumes, refined industrial seed oils, sugar, alcohol, and fun for thirty days. After the first hellish week, I turned the corner. My body felt amazing in every way and I had unlimited energy for the first time in my life. Every issue that I had started to slowly reverse itself. I could stay awake past 10pm. My chronic back, neck and joint pain lessened, and I was thrilled when my acne improved. My mood and outlook became endlessly positive. My skin glowed and my eyes were a bright white. I felt on top of the world and there was no way I was going back!

I kept up this way of eating and just kept improving. The more changes that I made, the better I felt and the more excited I was to continue to make even better choices. When I accidentally had even a sliver of gluten or corn, I felt absolutely awful. It was so pronounced that I've strictly been off gluten and most grains for years now. I don't miss them at all because I now know how they make me feel. Now I follow a modified Paleo-style diet, eating mostly whole, unprocessed foods that have been around since before the modern agricultural movement. I focus on adding in lots of veggies and eating the right kinds of local and ethically raised protein. Ancient and completely unmodified foods have been the most healing for me. Through experimentation, I have figured out which foods work best for me and which trigger skin breakouts. Though your trigger foods will be unique to you, here are mine (which are very common) to help you get started.

Gluten and Grains

Unfortunately, lots of foods contain gluten since it's one of the most commonly used food additives. This pesky little protein found in wheat, barley, rye, kamut, spelt, bulgur and more is often cross-contaminated in grains like oats or rice. More and more people are finding that taking gluten out of their diet results in major improvements. It is shocking just how many different problems it can cause.

Gluten is extremely difficult for everybody to digest, not just for people with celiac disease or gluten sensitivities. The gluten protein molecule is large and challenging to break down. Further, grains contain substances called antinutrients which block the absorption of other nutrients in your system. So when you look at a loaf of whole grain, "heart healthy" bread at the store and see a bunch of vitamins, minerals, and protein in the nutritional information—think again. The actual nutritional benefits are misleading. You may very well be missing out on absorbing other nutrients from any whole foods in your digestive tract.

The size of the gluten molecule alone can damage your gut and the villi on the walls of your intestines. Intestinal villi are tiny fingerlike projections that absorb food's nutrients for use by your body. If your villi are damaged, you are no longer able to fully absorb and use nutrients from the foods you eat—that is, until you heal your gut. Gluten can also cause leaky gut syndrome when the continual damage to your intestinal walls from your food has caused some of its layers to become permeable. This allows undigested food particles to get into your bloodstream, throwing your immune system into overdrive by trying to neutralize the foreign invaders. When your immune system is overstimulated and stressed, it then starts to attack the body's own healthy cells too, resulting in autoimmune disorders and systemic inflammation—including acne, which is skin inflammation. It's critically important to address your body's gut and any overall inflammation, and the first place to start is with your food.

Gluten was a major contributor to my acne and overall health problems and, for years, I had no clue. A reaction I had after eating even the tiniest amount of gluten was immediate, extreme exhaustion. It was so bad that I saw a doctor and tried to get into a sleep study to figure out why I was always tired. It would also make me breakout days later.

Refined Sugar

Refined sugar makes me breakout almost immediately and drastically affects my mood—no fun! White sugar, brown sugar and high fructose corn syrup all affect me. Sugars that I'm okay with are raw honey, molasses, Grade B maple syrup, real fruit juice and all fruits. So I have a lot of options when it comes to sweetness. I prefer to bake my own treats at home, but sometimes I'll try a gluten-free cupcake from a nice bakery. A helpful strategy for me has been adopting the mindset that the treat has to be worth it. If I try a dessert and it's less than amazing, I don't finish it or just throw it away. It doesn't feel wasteful when I know the affects it could have. I have noticed, however, that my tolerance to the occasional sugary treat is getting better over time.

Alcohol

Last but not least, a common skin trigger for me is alcohol. We all know alcohol is toxic to the body and significantly taxes the liver, challenges your body's detoxification processes and dehydrates you. It also contains many problematic chemicals, additives and is broken down into sugar inside the body. Yes, even red wine has its problems though you've probably heard it can be healthy.

Even a small amount of alcohol made me breakout in the beginning, but it seemed to get better over time. It helps if I take a pharmaceutical grade vitamin C supplement and a glutathione product. (See the Resource Guide for where you can get these.) I also drink a lot of organic kombucha the next day which has an amazing effect on my skin and how I feel overall. If you're celebrating and you need options, organic and biodynamic wine seemed to be the easiest on me, or a clear alcohol distilled from fruit or potatoes, not from grain. Overall, alcohol is just a rare thing for me now because of how it makes me feel. When feeling good all the time becomes your new norm, anything that makes you feel less than great naturally becomes less appealing. You can definitely get there too!

That's it for my main triggers. Let's talk about a few more common foods that could be causing your problems.

Dairy and Caffeine

Dairy can be a big issue. The protein casein found in dairy can be problematic for many to digest, causing intestinal issues. If you have a reaction to dairy, it could also be causing leaky gut or any of the issues mentioned in the section on gluten. Dairy can create a lot of mucus and congestion in the body. It can slow down your lymph system and your digestion as well as create congestion on your face.

A lot of people can experience problems with too much caffeine as well which can cause inflammation. It can increase cortisol in your body, causing stress on your system. Caffeine also acts as a diuretic so if you're drinking more than 1-2 cups per day you can become very dehydrated. Try to drink at least 2 cups of water for every cup of coffee you have to prevent dehydration. Dehydration can result in challenges flushing toxins out of your body. If your skin is very inflamed, try phasing out coffee completely and opt for green tea which is slightly caffeinated, or caffeine-free herbal tea.

Healthy Foods For Your Skin

Now that you're probably thoroughly bummed out and wanting to know what in the world you can actually eat, let's talk about the wealth of good foods that support your skin. A helpful tip is to adopt a mindset change when it comes to food. A lot of clients say the words, "I can't" when it comes to food. I can't have this food, or I can't eat that food. It's a negative statement and you can actually have whatever foods you want. Instead, you choose not to have foods that harm you and you choose to focus on eating foods that nourish your body. Try to catch yourself and make sure you use this little positive language trick. You can do whatever you want, whether its eating poorly or healthfully and you alone deal with the consequences of both. How you choose to live your life has been and will always be your choice. Stay empowered.

Vegetables and Fruits

Eat an unlimited amount of vegetables and constantly think about adding more. Get as many green leafy veggies into your meals as possible. Try making vegetables the base of your meals. Whether it's eating a salad, baking spaghetti squash, mashing up sweet potatoes or eating more stir-fry, you'll find endless tips and recipes online. Make this fun by going to the farmers market and picking out fresh, brightly colored vegetables. Add in healthy whole fats, herbs and spices to make your veggies taste good to you. High quality olive oil and sea salt taste great over many cooked vegetables. If you're not a vegetable fan, start slowly and try making homemade sauces and dressings like pesto, fresh vinaigrettes, or guacamole. Whatever you need to do to get more veggies in is fine. Carrot fries, zucchini noodles and sautéed spinach are some of my favorite ways to add in veggies.

Eat any kind of fruit you like but try and keep it to 1-2 servings per meal. Colorful berries give you the most nutritional bang for your buck and the lowest sugar content. Vary your fruits so you're not just eating tropical varieties like mango, pineapple or banana. Some nutrition experts get very specific about the sugar content in fruit but if you're starting from a standard diet, fruit is always a better choice than processed food. Just don't go on an all fruit binge. Dried fruits are okay in moderation and as snacks, just be cognizant of the higher sugar content. I love dried dates (not to be confused with figs or prunes which taste very different) as an occasional sweet snack. They're like nature's candy!

Nuts and Seeds

While most nuts and seeds are very nutritious, I don't recommend peanuts. Peanuts are often contaminated with mold and contain aflatoxin, a known carcinogen. Be careful and pay attention as sometimes people with major gut issues can be sensitive to nuts and/or seeds, but not always. You just have to experiment. Always opt for raw and organic whenever possible and experiment with new kinds you haven't tried before. Some of my favorites are brazil nuts, hazelnuts, pine nuts, cashews, pecans, walnuts, hemp seeds, sunflower seeds and sprouted chia seeds. Go to the health food store and browse the many options.

For other forms of healthy fats and snacks, I love any form of coconut (depending on who you ask, it can also be classified as a fruit). You can try unsweetened dried coconut flakes/shreds or coconut manna/coconut butter (which is great on a baked sweet potato with cinnamon and sea salt).

Dairy Alternatives

Substitute dairy or soy milk with coconut milk, almond milk, hemp milk, hazelnut milk or any other nut milk you can find. Read the label to make sure it doesn't contain added sugar or other processed ingredients. For cooking or smoothies, I use Living Harvest Tempt's Unsweetened Vanilla Hemp Milk or Pacific Foods' Organic Unsweetened Almond Milk since both have a neutral taste.

Coconut milk is by far my favorite dairy alternative. Coconut oil, found in the milk, has many positive health benefits and when ingested is antimicrobial, antiviral, antibacterial and antifungal, which supports your health and skin from the inside out.

Canned coconut milk has the cleanest ingredients and is the only way I buy it. Make sure you get the whole, unprocessed option, not the low fat one since processing it removes many of the amazing health benefits of whole coconut. The cleanest brands I've found include Thai Kitchen, Native Forest, Natural Value, or Whole Foods' 365 Brand. I like Natural Value since its cans do not contain BPA, a known hormone disruptor that does not help your body or skin. You can also make your own coconut milk by following one of the many recipes online.

You can also use coconut cream or coconut oil in place of coffee creamer. I like the Native Forest brand for coconut cream and Tropical Traditions, Carrington Farms or Artisana brands for coconut oil.

Animal Protein

High quality animal protein was a crucial part of regaining my health and can be a very healing food. Organic, grass-fed, free-range, pastured, and truly locally sourced is best. Protein is a health necessity, especially collagen and gelatin, in order to rebuild your intestinal lining if you have any kind of damage or leaky gut/autoimmune issues. You also need protein and collagen to repair damaged skin. However, don't overdo it and eat only meat like some recent diet trends might tell you to do. Meat is not a "free food" or one to consistently overindulge in. Animal protein is acidic to the body and having the right internal balance between acid and alkaline turns on your body's innate healing mechanisms. (Check out alkaline diets or alkaline water, but know they're not a long term solution.) Learn about and have fun visiting your local farms or go to Whole Foods or a health food store to find the best quality meat.

To give you some ideas, I eat 100% grass-fed beef, organic pastured local chicken, pastured local eggs, lamb, sheep, goat, pork, and local and sustainable fish. Find out what is available to you as locally as possible. I also experimented with organ meats, which are the nutritional superfoods of the animal, making a lot of high quality bone broth (see recipe in the Gut Healing Superfoods section). Organ meats (liver, kidney, etc.) can be amazing but they need to be prepared in a way that is as tasty as possible because they can taste very strange at first. Food is meant to taste good so, as a rule of thumb, high quality bacon fat and organic ghee helps everything taste better!

High Quality Fats

Use cold-pressed, unrefined, unheated olive, flax seed, coconut and avocado oils. Finding the best olive oil brand is especially important because there are many oils sold that are actually blended with rancid industrial seed oils, like canola. The high heat used to process canola destroys the oil's structure and creates free radicals and inflammation in your body. Canola oil is far from a skin supporting food.

True olive oil should produce a peppery bite at the back of your throat after you swallow it and almost make you cough. I love Bragg's Olive Oil or the affordable, widely available California Olive Ranch (which I recently saw at Target). Specialty olive oil shops are popping up everywhere and will often offer tastes.

Organic, grass fed ghee is another great high quality fat. Ghee is clarified butter often used in Indian cooking and does not contain the milk proteins that so many people struggle with. However, it still has a nice buttery taste and is full of skin supporting nutrients. So if dairy bothers you and you want to get the flavor of butter, try some ghee. It also has a high smoke point for cooking which means it's stable and doesn't cause free radicals or inflammation in the body like many other oils with a low smoke point. (Animal foods have much higher smoke points in general than other forms of oil, like olive oil.) Pure Indian Foods Organic Grass Fed Ghee is my favorite in both quality and flavor.

Sugar Alternatives

You can use any number of natural sweeteners, but keep this in mind: sugar is still sugar, and your body isn't designed for massive, unlimited quantities of sugar, natural or not. A lot of people with acne find that refined sugar is the biggest trigger for outbreaks. If you eat your sugar with fiber—in the form of real fruit—sugar more slowly absorbs into your bloodstream, which is less taxing on your body. A sudden rush of the sweet stuff will spike your insulin, often resulting in breakouts, not to mention weight gain. Think of insulin as the key that unlocks the door for fat to enter your cells.

Honey, maple syrup and molasses are my favorite options and, unlike processed sugar, they all have health boosting benefits. You can enjoy these unprocessed sweeteners in moderation.

Honey can be an incredible health food when used in moderation. It is the only food that naturally preserves itself forever. (Thanks, honeybees!) Raw, unfiltered, unprocessed honey is my favorite. It contains vitamins, enzymes, antioxidants, has antiviral and antibacterial properties, and aids healthy digestion. Local honey is best and you can often find it at your local health food store, farmers market or Whole Foods. Make sure you never feed honey to any infant under the age of one and if you are allergic to bees, ask your doctor before consuming honey as it could cause anaphylaxis.

Grade B maple syrup is less filtered and processed than Grade A and contains a higher mineral content. If the label doesn't say what grade it is, it's likely Grade A, and you should keep looking. Grade B maple syrup is full of minerals—zinc, magnesium, potassium, manganese, iron and calcium.

Real blackstrap molasses is chock full of minerals that support your skin like Vitamin B6, potassium, magnesium and manganese. While it's not always the most versatile sweetener, it's wonderful for baked goods, especially around the holidays.

Elimination Diet

Now that you have some new skin supporting food options to try, the next step is to embark on an elimination diet to determine your potential food triggers. Here's the basics of how it will work.

For twenty-one days, you will eliminate common trigger and allergen foods including grains, dairy, legumes, sugar, alcohol, soy, peanuts and refined oils. Instead, focus on the skin supporting foods we just reviewed like lots of vegetables, fruits, animal protein, high quality fat, dairy alternatives, nuts, seeds, and moderate amounts of sugar alternatives. There is no one way of eating so find what works best for you. You'll be amazed how much you can tell how food affects you once you take out the allergens. See my favorite cookbooks and blogs for inspiration in the Resource Guide.

On the 22nd day, reintroduce gluten-containing grains at each meal and see how you feel. Only reintroduce gluten and be careful to not reintroduce any of the other foods you took out at this time. You could have a bagel at breakfast, a sandwich at lunch, and some pasta with your dinner. Write down how you feel: Did you bloat? Any digestive distress? Do you feel cranky? Tired? Did you breakout? Any allergy like symptoms—runny nose, sneezing, etc.? Did you have more joint pain or headaches? If you had a reaction, take gluten back out and eat following the elimination diet for another 2-3 days to clear this reaction from your system.

Once you feel good again, try dairy. Drink some milk with breakfast, have some Greek yogurt (without added sugar) at lunch, and eat some cheese with dinner. Ask yourself the same questions and take an inventory of how you feel. If you have a reaction, take dairy out for 3 days again to clear your system.

Now, if you drank regularly before doing the elimination diet, try the same method with alcohol. Have a drink with dinner, trying anything other than beer which contains gluten. If you reacted to adding gluten back in, then it's best to stay away from grain alcohols during this test so you know the true effect of the alcohol and not any cross reaction from gluten. Then, pay attention the next day, doing an internal inventory again to see how you feel. If you feel awful and bloated, wait a few more days to clean your system out and then add sugar.

Sugar is often in foods with gluten or dairy, so make sure you know how you react to those two first. If you react poorly to both gluten and dairy, then in order to get an accurate sugar test, drink sugary soda, eat candy—or things that are just pure sugar.

Otherwise you won't really know how it affects you as clearly.

After testing sugar, follow the same process for soy and legumes. You can then try refined vegetable oils like canola, and then peanuts. However, I don't recommend either peanuts or refined oils even if they don't cause a reaction. You just want to get clear about your trigger foods so you know what you need to adamantly avoid in your diet.

Pay close attention to your skin and digestion throughout this entire process. Write everything down to keep track of your triggers, then apply what you learn to your life and watch it change!

Gut Healing Superfoods

If you had digestive reactions while adding foods back in, had digestive distress before doing the elimination diet, or noticed clearer skin during the 21 days, you'll want to focus on repairing your gut, which may be compromised in multiple ways.

Regular digestion is critically important for your skin. If you have problems with regular, easy elimination, toxic material sits in your intestines too long. This can cause the toxins to be reabsorbed through your intestinal walls and back into your bloodstream. Your breakouts could be caused by your body trying to detox through the skin since the digestive system is weak.

Healthy digestion means easily going to the bathroom 1-2 times per day. Any less than that and you could become cranky, anxious, depressed, irritable, and just generally feel toxic. Pay attention to how your digestion correlates with your skin. Work on repairing your digestion and making sure you are regular. A few tablespoons of virgin organic coconut oil aids digestion as does drinking a cup of warm lemon water in the morning.

Gelatin

I noticed a big difference when I added grass-fed gelatin to my diet. It's now one of my favorite gut superfoods. Gelatin is an animal protein that's easily digestible and helps repair your intestines. High in collagen, it has amazing beauty benefits and helps your skin repair faster and look younger. It also helps with any knee and joint pain.

Try a tablespoon of grass-fed gelatin in the morning and at night. Great Lakes makes a high quality grass-fed gelatin that will solidify into gel or gummies and a collagen hydrolysate that is cold water soluble and even easier to digest. Be sure to clean your utensils with warm water and soap immediately after using gelatin—it can be a huge pain to clean once it has solidified. The cold soluble gelatin is great for traveling because you can put it in anything to get in your dose.

I slowly pour the grass-fed gelatin powder into my tea or coffee while stirring to prevent clumping which is important because it gels easily. Working with gelatin can take a little getting used to. When I use it in my coffee, I also add coconut oil and cinnamon so it doesn't make me crave sugar or crash. Sometimes I drink Dave Aspery's Bulletproof coffee (found on the Bulletproof Executive website). Be sure to pay attention to how caffeine affects you. If you are a frequent caffeine consumer, it could cause challenges with your skin.

Bone Broth

Traditional bone broth is another amazing gut healing and skin superfood. It's the easily digestible base of many ancient healing soups that is made from scratch. Bone broth has a lot of the same benefits as gelatin but it's important that you know the source of the bones you are using. If you're making beef broth, the bones should come from 100% grass-fed, hormone-free, and ethically raised animals. If you're making chicken broth, the chickens should be pastured. Find a local source for chicken bones or ask questions at your health food store. Whole Foods can help you determine the quality of the animal. Use this basic recipe to make bone broth.

Bone Broth Recipe

3 medium-large carrots

3 celery stalks

1 small-medium onion

2 pounds beef, chicken, or fish bones

1-2 cloves garlic, crushed

1 tablespoon Celtic sea salt

2 tablespoons apple cider vinegar

Purified water

1. Roughly chop the carrots, celery and onion and put into a crockpot.

2. Place the bones on top.

3. Add the garlic, sea salt and apple cider vinegar.

4. Fill to the top with purified water.

5. Cook on low for 10-18 hours.

6. Once cool, strain through a colander and throw away the bones and vegetable scraps.

Try to drink a warm cup of bone broth daily, adding Celtic sea salt for taste and extra minerals. Use the broth as a base to make delicious soup with whatever vegetables or meat you like. Pay attention to how your skin looks after you've been drinking your homemade broth for a week.

Supplements

My experience with supplements is that it's best to obtain your nutrients from whole, high quality, organic foods. We are only beginning to understand the many nutrients contained in food and how they interact with each other in order for our bodies to utilize their full benefit. So, for a nutrient rich diet, try to eat a rainbow of vegetables, brightly colored berries, organic, ethically raised, high quality animal products and healthy, whole, unrefined fats. You have to eat anyway, so why not get your supplements free through your food!

That said, a few supplements can be beneficial to speed your healing. One of my favorites is Natural Calm—a magnesium supplement taken at night. It helps you sleep, reduces stress and promotes healthy digestion. I also like digestive enzymes like Rainbow Light's Advanced Enzyme System which helps your body break down food.

If you're looking for extra help with digestion or just want to step up your skin supporting efforts, I recommend adding probiotic supplements. I like the brands Seeking Health ProBiota Bifido (which is dairy free), Bio-Kult, Prescript-Assist, and Garden of Life Primal Defense. Try one brand at a time and see how you do.

I also like fish oil supplements which benefit your skin and overall health. It's important to buy a high quality filtered fish oil since mercury pollution is a real problem now in fish. Green Pastures' fermented Cinnamon Tingle cod liver oil is one of the easiest ways to add fish oil to your diet and definitely the best tasting. Their oil is obtained through the traditional method of fermentation which keeps nutrients from being destroyed during the process. Or, you can try flax oil which is easier for your body to process. Barlean's makes great flavored flax oils.

Biotin is another favorite supplement of mine that helps with skin regeneration, nail strength and hair growth. I take one Seeking Health's Biotin 5 daily.

Other Ways to Support the Gut and Digestion

- Add olive oil to everything you can—cooked veggies, soups, salads. Real extra virgin olive oil tastes wonderful and I never knew this until I had some. The imposters don't even come close. Adding extra virgin olive oil and Celtic sea salt is my go-to for quickly and easily improving taste.

- Drink plenty of water and fluids. Add lemon, lime, mint, raspberries, pineapple—whatever you can to make it more appealing. For carbonation, try San Pellegrino, Perrier, or another natural sparkling mineral water. If you drink a lot of coffee or soda, start by gradually swapping out a glass of water in their place. Then, gradually increase your intake so you are drinking mostly water all day long.

- Eat the rainbow, adding as many colorful fruits and veggies as you can to cleanse your system and keep your skin clear. Eating raw fruits and vegetables is another great way to get more water into your system. You can also make smoothies or juice, just remember to drink them over a 20 minute period to minimize any blood sugar spikes.

- Sleep. Sleep. Sleep. It is so important for everything— your skin will heal faster, your digestion will be better, and your mood will be more positive. You will make better food choices because your body won't be run down and craving energy or sugar. It's also an important factor in maintaining a healthy weight. To help with sleep:

- Keep as consistent a bedtime as possible and incorporate a ritual, like lighting candles, drinking tea (try Traditional Medicinals Nighty Night, chamomile, or lavender tea), or reading a book if it makes you sleepy.

- Take a relaxing bath before bed with some magnesium crystals.

- Try a nightly magnesium supplement, like that made by Natural Calm.

- Spray your pillow with diluted lavender essential oil or other sleep blends made of essential oils.

- To help your body's natural rhythms, turn down the lights, lighting candles instead. Watch less TV and do your best to stay off the computer.

- Make your room as dark as possible, covering any light coming from the TV, clocks or radios. Wear a comfortable sleep mask to block out the light.

- Get blackout curtains. So amazing!

- Try a noise machine or any other white noise. (I bought one from Bed, Bath & Beyond for about $20 that plays the sounds of the ocean, breezes and rivers.) Or download a free app on your phone.

- Figure out a temperature that works for you, then stick with it. (Though sleeping in a cooler room is great for most, I need to be warm in order to fall asleep so I say to just figure out what works for you.)

- Invest in bedding that you love to make your bed a comforting place. If you like your sheets to feel cool, buy ones made of soft, crisp fabric. If you like warmth, get some flannel sheets.

- Just being outdoors and the sun both help with sleep. Take a relaxing walk through nature whenever you can. Find some form of outdoor exercise you love, especially since exercise improves sleep too. Fresh air also helps with detoxing. And, it's free!

If you do all of the simple things above and still need more, here are some additional methods to try.

1. Try a sleep induction mat or any acupressure mat. It takes some getting used to and is slightly uncomfortable, but it will knock you out in about 10-20 minutes. It also helps with back pain and circulation.

2. Try Earthing. You know how good it feels when you're at the beach or walking around barefoot all day? Well, there's more to it than just relaxing. Turns out that when our bare skin is in direct contact with the Earth, the ground pulls free electrons out of our bodies. It's referred to as either Earthing and grounding. I have experienced deeper sleep, faster muscle recovery, and an overall reduction in pain by using a grounding mat and grounding bed sheet. Earthing is free and easy when weather permits and you can walk or sit outside.

3. On your computer a lot? I use tinted computer glasses made by Gunnar Optiks. They keep the screen's blue light from interfering with circadian rhythms and help reduce eye strain from long stints on the computer.

7

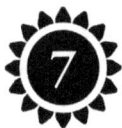

Reducing Toxicity

Lately, we have been bombarded with messages about detoxes and cleanses and the need for cleaning up our internal environment. In an industrialized world, we breathe, eat, and literally bathe in chemicals. Our bodies are smart and efficient and they process these chemicals as foreign invaders, going on the defensive to clean them out in the kidneys and liver. But, sometimes the workload of this bogs down our bodies.

There's a huge connection for a lot of people between the liver and the skin. The largest detox organ, the skin removes toxins from the body. While we clean up our food, we see faster results by helping the body naturally detox some of the junk we're carrying around.

Here are some of my favorite daily detox strategies.

Oil Pulling

This ancient Ayurvedic healing method pulls toxins out of your bloodstream by way of your mouth. It whitens your teeth and freshens your breath. It's helped not just the overall health of my mouth but with my acne, allergies, and congestion too. My holistic dentist has noticed a difference and even the dental hygienist comments on my healthy gums and white teeth. It continues to deliver a lot of results for me. Try it for a week and see what you notice.

How to Do It

Drink a glass of water upon waking up. On an empty stomach, before you shower or brush your teeth, put about 1 tablespoon of coconut oil or sesame oil in your mouth and "chew" until it melts. (It's important to note that research on oil pulling used sesame oil. However, I have had the same success with coconut oil.) The oil will take about 10 seconds to melt. Keeping your mouth closed, swish the oil through your mouth, gently "pulling" it back and forth between your teeth. Keep it away from the back of your throat to avoid gagging. Do this for about 20 minutes then spit out the oil into the garbage, never the sink, to avoid clogging. Follow this by rinsing your mouth with water and brushing your teeth really well to remove all the toxins from your mouth. I know, it sounds like a long time, but you can do it while in the shower or bathroom, or before anyone else in your family wakes up. If you only have 5 or 10 minutes, that's okay too.

Tongue Scraping

Here's a little trick to maximize your oil pulling's effectiveness—the tongue scraper! It's quick, easy, and inexpensive. A tongue scraper literally scrapes away any debris and buildup off of your tongue, resulting in a super clean mouth with extra fresh breath. Scrapers are much more effective than brushing your tongue. They are inexpensive and found at most health food stores. I have a simple copper metal one that scrapes well and can be cleaned easily.

How to Do It

Either first thing in the morning or at night while brushing your teeth, gently glide the scraper across your tongue and rinse off the residue. Do this a few times with good pressure, being careful not to scrape your taste buds or cause any bleeding. Rinse and repeat 5-10 times. Do this once and you'll likely be hooked—and disgusted by what came off of your tongue.

Dry Body Brushing

This technique feels wonderful. Dry body brushing is an Ayurvedic technique with many skin and overall health benefits. It's an inexpensive daily detox strategy that boosts your circulation and gets your lymph moving. It removes dead skin cells and encourages new skin to emerge. It helps with body blemishes and those pesky keratin deposits on your arms we call "chicken skin," as well as opens your pores to release toxins. Some have found it improves the appearance of cellulite (not that any of you beautiful creatures have that unsightly stuff).

All you need is a dry body brush. (I use the Yerba Prima Tampico Skin Brush found on Amazon.) Clean the brush with warm water, gentle castile soap, and tea tree essential oil.

A few general rules before you get started:

- Brush toward your heart to help with circulation and bringing lymph back to your heart. Around your stomach, brush in a clockwise circular motion to help with digestion. Also, brush in a circular motion around joints like elbows and knees.

- Do not brush on broken skin, scabs or very sensitive skin. Do not brush on varicose veins. And never dry brush your face. Ouch! Your skin should be pink afterward, not red or irritated.

- The thinner the skin, the lighter the pressure. Go crazy on the bottoms of your feet, but be gentle on the tops.

- Use long sweeping motions. Think about helping your lymph move and stimulating circulation through your body with the brush.

Go over each area 3-5 times, or use 3-5 long, sweeping brush strokes.

How to Do It

Start at the bottoms of your feet. Brush starting at your toes going toward the bottoms of your heels. Then do the same over the tops of your feet, but don't press quite as hard on this thinner skin.
Now, brush up both legs. Start wherever, just use long, upward strokes. (I usually go from my ankles to my knees 3-5 times on the front of my legs and then the same on the back.) Use the same long, upward strokes from your knees to your thighs, front and back.

Concentrate some extra love wherever you may have some cellulite: thighs, legs, butt. Go for it! Then on to your glutes—brush in long, upward strokes again 3-5 times per cheek. Brush your whole stomach in circular motions, and then focus a little extra time on your lower abs.

For your back, think about where your heart is. Start at your mid-back and brush up toward your heart and stop there. For your upper back, brush down toward your heart and stop around your shoulders.

For women, brush in gentle circular motions around your chest, going around each pec separately in a circular motion. Be careful: this skin is sensitive. For men, brush straight toward your heart since you likely have nothing in the way. (And for the approximately 5% of readers who are male, thanks for being here. Love you!)

Now, treat your hands just like your feet. Brush the palms starting at your fingertips and go all the way up the bottom side of your arm to your elbows or armpits. Do the back of your hands, starting at your fingertips, and brush all the way over the tops of your arms up to your shoulders.

For armpits, brush gently down toward your heart. Brush the back of your neck carefully, and generally don't brush the thin, sensitive skin on the front.

Total time brushing should be about 5 minutes, though you can go up to 20 minutes if you really want to feel great. Breathe deeply and make it a relaxing ritual. Then, jump in the shower or bath—your pores will be open and ready to detox the junk out.

Toxicity & Your Home Environment

You may not think of your home as something that adds to your toxic load but it is likely full of indoor air pollutants. We spend so much time indoors that cleaning up the air in our home is really important. Many things in our homes leak gas or seep chemical and plastic residues into the air—the paint on the walls, the flame retardants on the mattress or couch, the chemicals in household cleaners, and the electromagnetic frequencies (EMFs) emitted from computers, TVs, and cell phones. Whatever you breathe in, your body must neutralize and process, adding to its overall burden and taking energy away from its ability to cleanse and heal. How can we combat these toxic items in our modern lives? Making simple switches result in big changes.

Indoor Plants

Indoor plants are great for filtering indoor air and improving air quality. I love ivy, vines, prayer lilies, and anything else beautiful. Ask your local nursery to recommend sturdy, indoor plants (which is helpful if you're not a great gardener). Google "NASA Clean Air Study" for more suggestions.

Let Nature Indoors

I know this is obvious, but if weather permits, open the windows, the patio door, or the shades. Do whatever you can to get more outside air and light into your space. You'll notice a huge lift in your energy and mood.

Beeswax Candles

Pure beeswax candles are a great addition to your home. Big Dipper makes beautiful ones. Beeswax is the only candle wax that actually filters out and improves air quality. If you can't find beeswax or it's too expensive, opt for palm wax or soy wax with natural scents. Know that beeswax burns a lot longer as well. If you're up for it, get creative by making your own candles—melt the wax and add a few drops of essential oil.

Himalayan Rock Salt Lamps

Himalayan rock salt lamps or candle holders are another inexpensive way to improve indoor air quality. They emit negative ions and counteract EMF indoor air pollution. Place lamps or candle holders where you spend a lot of time or close to your electronics to combat the EMFs. Their range is limited so make sure they are relatively close by.

Indoor Air Filters

Indoor air filters are another way to dramatically improve your indoor air quality. These are separate, standalone units, not the ones you already have in the walls of your apartment or home. (However, you should make sure you change those filters frequently.) They can be expensive, but you'll want one with a HEPA filter that also emits negative ions. Dr. Mercola sells a good one on his health website which is listed in the Resource Guide. It may even help with seasonal allergies and respiratory issues.

Get Outside

Going outside for a walk each day will not only get you fresh air but also help your stress levels. Nature's sights and sounds reduce stress and breathing fresh air and getting sunshine will help your sleep. A big misconception is that the sun is not good for your skin but Vitamin D is important to your overall health, and sunlight has powerful natural disinfectant properties.

I highly recommend using only natural sun protectant instead of chemical laden commercial sunscreen. Wear hats and clothing to protect from overexposure. Or, apply coconut oil to your body. It has a low natural SPF of about 8. Implementing just a short daily walk can be a dramatic game changer. Go outside even if only for a 20 minute walk. Be creative in getting more time outside. Your body will thank you.

Natural Household Cleaners

I'm so happy that I made the switch to all natural, basic products a few years ago. It was a lot of work in the beginning trying to figure out which products and DIY recipes work, but it was definitely worth it. Remember that everything you do for your body is a gift worth giving.

Here are some simple products you can buy that really work. If interested in more, you can find a lot of DIY natural home cleaning recipes online that call for simple ingredients like baking soda, vinegar, washing soda, and essential oils. Those four will get you a lot of mileage in your home and they're inexpensive.

1. Dr. Bronner's Sal Suds is a highly concentrated all-purpose home cleaner. I use it as dish soap: mix it with water (about 1

part soap to 4 parts water) and a few drops of orange, lemon, or lemongrass essential oil, then store in a glass bottle with a pour spout on top. It's also a great liquid laundry detergent.

2. Dr. Bronner's Castile Soap can be diluted with 3 parts water for use on your face or any laundry requiring hand washing. It's also a great all-purpose soap.

3. Eco Nuts and Nellies All Natural Laundry Soaps are hypo allergenic and great for sensitive skin. For a natural lightening agent or extra cleaning power, use Charlie's Soap Oxygenated Bleach. Pretreat using Grandma's Laundry Stain Stick or just a drop of lemon essential oil to remove stains, letting it soak in. Be sure to spot test first!

4. Instead of dryer sheets, use organic cotton wool balls (and a lavender sachet if you want to add a scent). The wool stops static cling and reduces drying time. Plus, they last a very long time.

5. Use plain white vinegar and newspaper for cleaning windows and mirrors. You may need to try it a few times to remove any residue left by conventional window cleaners.

6. Microfiber cleaning cloths can be used for dusting without a spray or anything else, and they last a long time.

7. It's easy to make your own all-purpose kitchen or bathroom cleaner with citrus fruits like lemon, lime, or orange. Throw citrus peels in a bag in the freezer until you have enough to fill a mason jar, then put the peels in a jar to the top, sprinkle with sea salt, and fill with vinegar. Close the jar tightly, shake, and then leave on the counter, preferably in a sunny spot, for four to six weeks. Once done, shake the jar and pour the solution into a bottle with a spray top until halfway full. Mix with water, shake, and you're all set. This is a potent degreaser and I love the citrus germ killing power.

8.   Baking soda with a mixture of essential oils will do the trick for many other household needs. (I mix mine with tea tree, lavender, and orange oils for the bathroom.) Sprinkle the baking soda onto whatever surface you're cleaning and spray with vinegar. Then, let the two do their magic for about 10 minutes or so. Come back and scrub or wipe clean.

9.   Branch Basics is a gentle, amazing all-around natural home cleaner. I'm not sure there's anything it can't clean.

As you buy cleaning solutions for your home, opt for simple ingredients that you know. Experiment to find solutions to any problems you might have. For example, my natural laundry soap didn't leave my clothes with any fragrance, so I did some research and found that I could just put a few drops of lemon essential oil in the load. Not only did my clothes smell fresh but the oil also fights stains. If your family's resistant to making changes, explain that you're putting in the work to heal, and your health is a top priority. Or, you can always do laundry separately for a while until your family is on board.

....

Invest in Essential Oils

High quality essential oils can seem expensive, but you need only a few types to get started with cleaning. My favorites are tea tree and lemon which are powerful germ and virus killers. Or, go crazy with eucalyptus and lavender which have the same fighting power as tea tree and lemon. If you pick only one, choose lavender—it is the most versatile. Simple and powerful!

....

KATHERINE LARSEN

8

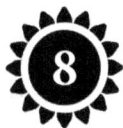

Attitude of Gratitude

For a few years, I did everything right—used super skin supporting products for my skin, got enough rest, drank water, detoxed, almost always ate clean—but my skin still had significant challenges. Although my breakouts were smaller and easier to hide, I stressed over them. I examined my face every day, cursing my skin for betraying me. Then, I read a book on gratitude.

I began to practice gratitude in many areas of my life. My skin was one of my first areas of focus. I chose to be grateful daily for the skin I had, even though I knew deep inside that I was far from happy with it. I focused on the small patches of my face that were smooth. I noticed a healthy glow, even through the acne. Noticing these things made me see my skin differently. Nothing changed at first but I felt more beautiful when I looked in the mirror.

I lavished my skin with love and I was gentler with it. I took time with my skincare routine in the morning and night. I no longer rushed through washing my face or applying moisturizer. I thanked my skin for all the work that it does for me every day—sometimes silently, other times out loud like a crazy person, which was very fun. I appreciated when it was tan, when it was pale, when it was red, and even when it was tired. I thanked my skin for telling me that something wasn't right inside my body.

Amazing changes started to happen. I stopped trying so hard, I used fewer products, I fell asleep without washing my face at night, and I indulged in the occasional glass of wine. I found that none of these things had any effect on my skin. In fact, my skin got better despite relaxing my routine. To me, it felt like a miracle, especially after all the work to find the perfect routine and formula for my face.

Let me help you appreciate your skin too. Your skin is completely unique: the color, the texture, the tone, each mole and freckle is entirely yours. No one looks exactly like you so try enjoying and celebrating your unique features. I used to hate how my eyes would squint when I smiled. Now I've learned to embrace and be grateful for having such a joyful expression.

Your skin is an amazing barrier that keeps you safe from the dangers and harms of the world outside your body's ecosystem. It heals itself, it regulates temperature, and it helps get rid of toxins. It's the only skin you have so start reminding yourself how incredible it is.

Here are some fun skin facts to jump start your skin appreciation:

1. Your skin is your body's largest organ.

2. Your skin renews itself every 28 days.

3. Your skin has its own bacteria microbiome of more than 1,000 species.

4. Your skin has natural fats that keep the outer layer nourished and healthy. Detergents and alcohol can destroy these lipids.

5. Every minute, your skin sheds 30,000 skin cells.

6. The thinnest skin in your body is your eyelids at only 0.02 millimeters thick.

Pretty amazing, huh? Now onto the daily gratitude practice that helped me so much. Every morning for 30 days, I wrote down a list of 10 things for which I was grateful. This started my day on an incredibly positive note and helped in many other areas of my life.

Make a list of 10 things such as:

1.   I am grateful that my skin allows me to feel all the joys of touch.

   a.   I am grateful my skin lets me feel my dog's soft fur.
   b.   I am grateful my skin lets me feel hugs from my loved ones.
   c.   I am grateful my skin helps me feel the sun's warmth.

2.   I am grateful my skin works so hard every day to keep me safe.

   a.   Thank you, skin, for fighting bacteria for me.
   b.   Thank you, skin, for automatically healing yourself.
   c.   Thank you, skin, for sending me messages when I'm too cold or hot.

First on my list, almost every day, I made sure to include, "Thank you for my beautiful, clear, youthful, glowing skin." Even if you don't believe it at first, keep saying it and you eventually will. The key is to focus on the positive—whatever it is. Anything can be reframed in a positive way. You're alive! Yes, you have acne, but you're alive!

Although it may seem silly, it really worked for me. Find parts of your body for which you are grateful: a freckle, or dimple, or a soft part of your skin. Maybe it's a smooth spot on your forehead, or that you're 40 and don't have many wrinkles around your eyes. Look hard and you will find multiple things. Always keep it positive and write it down.

Think hard about the things people often compliment you on. I once saw a young woman in New York City who had the most beautiful and interesting skin. She had dark hair, very pale pink skin, and light tan freckles covering her entire face. It is very hard to describe but her beautiful complexion looked like a painting. I would have never been compelled to say anything if I hadn't been through so much with my own skin. It is important to me that women know how gorgeous they are!

She was shy and uncomfortable when I told her how stunning and unique I found her skin. I asked her if people often complimented her skin and she sheepishly said, "Yes." I then asked if she believed them and she said, "Not really." I tell this story for all of you women out there who don't believe in your own beauty. If people compliment you for some trait you have, it's because it is truly beautiful.

We are conditioned to believe that we are never pretty or perfect enough. We are. Each one of us is a work of art. Believe you're beautiful and you will start to know it. Grasp onto that and don't let anyone take it from you. Tell yourself in the mirror today how wonderful you look, and tell your friends when they look good too. We get stronger by lifting up one another.

Say It Out Loud

Now that you've written your list, read each item out loud and say "thank you" three times. Do this every morning for at least 30 days and see what a difference it makes. If your skin heals, start being grateful for other areas of your life: family, love, career, nature, joy, health, pets, music. There is so much to be grateful for.

Before you go to bed, say out loud (or in your mind) 3 things for which you are grateful. Since we're focusing on skin, make them

3 things about your skin for that day. You can repeat some of the things you said in the morning but reflect on your day and try to find 3 experiences or moments during which you were grateful for your skin, or even your body. When you really think about everything our bodies do, the list is endless:

1. I am grateful that I felt the fresh air on my face.

2. I am grateful that my body protects me from illness every day.

3. I am grateful that my body keeps me warm.

4. I am grateful that my body allows me to dance, or run, or play sports.

5. I am grateful that my body allows me to sing, play music, play with my kids, or hug my friends.

After each of the 3 things, say "thank you" 3 times, just like you did in the morning. Make this a simple but important practice you do every night.

Another way to incorporate gratitude into your life is to say "thank you" in the mirror whenever you look at your face. You can say it to yourself: "Thank you, skin, you are perfect and healthy." When we suffer from skin conditions, it's easy to look in the mirror and feel frustration, anger, sadness, or low self-worth. You have to change that as soon as possible to truly heal. Find something to be grateful for, digging deeper each time. Do this every time you look in a mirror and it will soon become an ingrained practice.

When you are getting ready in the morning, showering, putting on lotion—this is a time to love your skin! Think about how you're nourishing your skin with your daily routine. Tell your skin it's worth it when you do a spot treatment or lavish on a serum. Slow down and learn to enjoy your routine, even if just for a minute.

When you just splash water on your face, say "thank you" to keep expressing gratitude for your skin. Pay attention to how this small change makes a huge impact on your life.

Notice you seem to be getting more attention? Are you receiving more compliments on your appearance? Be warned. Gratitude can often have that effect!

9

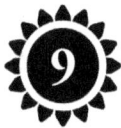

Implementing Powerful Skin Positivity

What you say about your skin can manifest into reality. This can be very difficult when we have a breakout. We're compelled to make excuses for it or we draw attention to it. When we draw attention to a blemish, we take the power away from anyone else who might criticize us for it.

Have you ever noticed how often you or others do this? Your best friend has a huge zit, which you can obviously see, but she still points it out anyway like it's the elephant in the room. Do you complain about your skin or talk about your acne? Stop it immediately—stop saying anything other than positive things about your skin right now. It will take practice, but start by not saying them aloud to others. Have you ever noticed that problems you dwell on seem to persist? Pretend your skin is beautiful and clear. Act as if you have perfect skin. Go to the party anyway, be confident, and make new friends. You'll send a powerful subconscious message to your body.

Here's one of my favorite positive thinking strategies: every time I catch myself thinking a negative thought about my skin or body, I stop. I reverse the thought and say something positive 3 times in my head (or, out loud, if I'm not in a place where people will think I've lost it). It's often as simple as, "I love you, body." "Thank you, body." "You work so hard to keep me healthy and safe every day and I appreciate it." I know, but just try it and see how different you will feel in your skin.

Pay attention to that running dialogue in your head and ask yourself whether the thoughts are healthy and positive. If it's anything less than good, reverse it. Go slow and don't get frustrated. Just remind yourself to add more positive statements than negative and eventually it will become natural to you. Remember, your skin is worth it!

Stress

Stress is potent. It releases the hormone cortisol into the body which quickly affects acne. I noticed that I was stressed all the time—constantly rushing through the day whether taking a shower, running errands, or working. I breathed and moved very quickly. Once I consciously made an effort to relax into what I was doing, I realized just how quickly and stressfully I was moving. I was able to become fully present. Using the following techniques, I can breathe deeply and slowly to relax.

The 4-7-8 Breath

One of my favorite ways to reduce stress is an ancient yoga breathing technique called the 4-7-8 Breath. (Dr. Andrew Weil has a great video on his website that can teach you about it.) It helps me fall asleep if I'm particularly stressed.

How to Do It

Touching the tip of your tongue to the tissue behind your teeth, breathe in through your nose deeply and slowly while you count to four. Hold your breath for seven counts, and then exhale audibly through your mouth for eight counts, making a whooshing sound. Pursing your lips helps. For the first month, do this cycle for no more than four times twice daily. After a month, you can do it up to eight cycles at a time. The 4-7-8 Breath powerfully reduces stress and anxiety.

Diaphragmatic or Low-Belly Breathing

While working toward healing, I noticed that every time I was stressed, worried or uncomfortable, my breath became shallow or erratic, or I found I was holding my breath without realizing it. I became aware, changed my breathing, and noticed a big difference in how I felt. I also felt more grounded. I do the following exercise whenever I feel stressed. When I'm with other people, they don't even notice I'm doing it.

How to Do It

Place a hand underneath your rib cage and a hand on your chest. Inhale deeply. Your chest and shoulders shouldn't move at all, only your stomach, so pay attention to the hand on your chest to determine if you're doing it correctly. Inhale deeply and feel your stomach expand slowly. Then, exhale slowly and feel it contract. Do this on a 3-5 second count each way to automatically calm your breathing.

Breathing Bonus

For you biohackers, techies, or interested people: HeartMath makes a great iPhone app and component that supports maximum relaxation in the body. Basically, you're optimizing your heartbeat to vary slightly in seconds between beats. HeartMath's sensors give you immediate feedback to help you breathe in a pattern that reduces stress and supports healing. It's about making sure you are in a specific heart rate variability zone, not just breathing slowly. I used mine for years, especially on planes during business travel. With practice, it's now much easier for me to get in the optimal zone without the device.

Emotional Freedom Technique (EFT) Tapping

EFT Tapping, also known as meridian tapping, was discovered in the late 1970s by a psychologist who was not making progress with a patient trying to get over a debilitating phobia. Part acupressure and part energy psychology, it has recently gained traction. Once you've tried it, you will be tapping with one hand on different meridian end points in your body while talking out loud. Yep, that's right.

I was skeptical about this approach but when you have nothing to lose, you'll try anything. I was amazed at how dramatically this technique immediately reduced my stress, cleared emotions and shifted my mindset. Whenever my stress spirals out of control, I do the tapping exercise for 5-10 minutes and instantly feel better. I think of it as reprogramming the software in my brain, or getting rid of the bugs.

Google "The Tapping Solution" for the science behind why it works. I also recommend reading The Tapping Solution by Nick Ortner. If you're struggling with weight, a must read is Tapping for Weight Loss and Body Confidence by Jessica Ortner. This brother-sister duo offers a lot of information and have worked hard to bring the results of this technique to the masses.

How to Do It

Rate how strong your emotions are surrounding your skin. Pick a phrase that feels true to you, like, "My acne is ruining my life" or, "I hate my skin." Then, on a scale of 1 to 10, rate how strong the emotion in that statement feels to you and write it down. If it's horrible and truly ruining your life, then the emotional charge is a 10. If it is sort of bothering you, then it's a 1.

Next, choose a setup statement. It can be something like, "Even though I have acne, I deeply and completely love and accept myself." Even if the statement doesn't feel real to you, say it anyway. If you can't say, "I love and accept myself," instead say, "It's okay for now." Just find a true statement about accepting yourself while also validating your feelings about your skin.

Now you will move onto the actual tapping. Using the fingertips of one hand, gently tap on the points of the body shown in the diagram below. Tap with equal pressure or roll through the fingertips, almost as if tapping your nails or fingers on a table.

First, tap lightly on the karate chop point. (We will use this point once at the start of the tapping session, when saying the setup statement out loud. You will tap through all the other points shown in the diagram in a cycle.) This point is located along the entire side of your palm, below your pinky. This is the edge of your hand that you see martial artists use to "chop" wooden planks or blocks. While tapping this point, say your setup statement 3 times: "Even though I have this acne, I deeply and completely love and accept myself."

Using the same tapping motion with your fingers, move through the tapping points on the body shown in the image, tapping on all the negative things you are feeling. This is your chance to vent, so say them all out loud.

The Body's Tapping Points

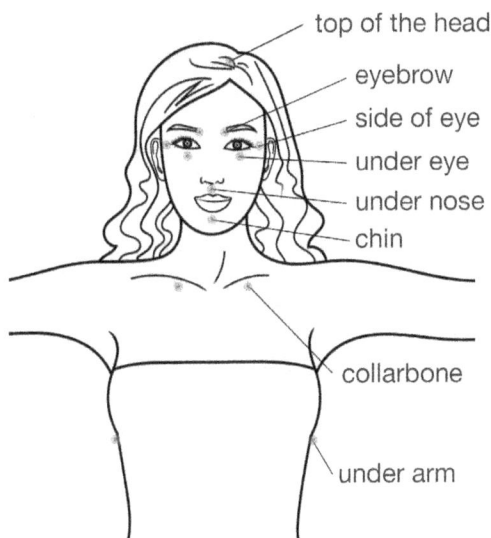

I'm including an example script below to get you started, but say whatever feels real to you. I initially had a hard time with this but this exercise won't affirm your negative beliefs—it just gives a voice to the toxic thoughts in your head in order to clear yourself of them holding you back. In this first part, make sure you stay on the negative thoughts to get everything out. You may feel overwhelmed with emotion. You may cry. It's okay. This is your time to heal. Get all the junk out.

1. Top of the head: I hate my skin.

2. Eyebrow: I feel so disgusting.

3. Side of the eye: My skin has betrayed me.

4. Under the eye: Why did this happen to me?

5. Under the nose: It's not fair.

6. Chin: Everybody is judging me. I can't even leave the house.

7. Collarbone: I'm so stressed out about my acne.

8. Under the arm: This is so embarrassing.

9. Top of the head: I can't take this acne anymore.

10. Eyebrow: I've had skin issues for so long and I'm so tired.

11. Side of the eye: I just want to disappear.

12. Under the eye: My skin hurts so badly.

13. Under the nose: How much longer until I find a cure?

14. Chin: I have tried everything!

15. Collarbone: I am so angry at my face.

16. Under the arm: I feel so helpless.

Notice when you start to feel some relief, maybe you've let out a sigh or tear up and feel a little calmer now. Whatever it is, as the negative emotion around your skin calms down, you can move on to the positive beliefs. Start this with a gentle suggestion and think of these positive statements as uploading new positive software into your brain. Again, say whatever feels good to you. I've found that sometimes when I have a hard time shifting into the positive statements, I can ask questions first. It's a subtle, gentle suggestion to get me to the place where I can feel positive.

I have also found it incredibly effective to combine the positive tapping statements with the gratitude concepts we discussed in the previous chapter. I'll tap on the points and say, "Thank you for my skin," or, "Thank you, skin, for keeping me healthy," or, "Thank you for my healing." The script below is to just give you ideas. Find what feels right and true to you, keeping it positive to reprogram your thoughts around your skin. If you find a particular phrase that resonates powerfully, keep tapping through the points, repeating that exact statement until you are ready to move to a new one.

1. Top of the head: My skin does so much for me.

2. Eyebrow: It works so hard every day.

3. Side of the eye: My skin protects me.

4. Under the eye: It keeps me healthy.

5. Under the nose: Maybe I can accept my skin.

6. Under the chin: Maybe it's not betraying me but helping me.

7. Collarbone: Today I choose to love my skin.

8. Under the arm: Thank you, skin.

9. Top of the head: I love you, skin.

10. Eyebrow: You are so beautiful.

11. Side of the eye: I am so healthy.

12. Under the eye: I am so grateful for my skin.

13. Under the nose: My skin is amazing.

14. Collarbone: My skin is clear.

Under the arm: My skin is perfect.

When you begin to feel relief, take a few slow, deep breaths. Measure the intensity of the statement you started with and see if your stress around your skin has lessened. Continue to tap with a new setup statement, or use the same one until you feel better. Try doing this daily for a week, anywhere between 5 and 15 minutes, and see how it affects you.

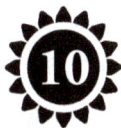

Travel Strategies

For years I traveled for work. I'd be gone for two or three days at a time, sometimes as long as five. I have lived all over the country and travel often to see friends and family. I noticed that travel tended to be a big breakout trigger for me, so I had to find ways to minimize it. This chapter is meant to help you travelers keep up your new routine while on the road.

First, here's what my travel kit looks like:

1. My pillowcase from home. I started doing this when I thought that the sheets or detergents may have been the cause of my breakouts. Once I realized that wasn't the case, I continued to pack it because it had a comforting effect.

2. Dry body brush. I like to do my dry body brushing ritual while I'm on the road. It helps my body detox and stay happy when I'm exposed to food and an environment that may not be the cleanest.

3. Asian Magic Exfoliating Square. When I travel, I rarely have access to an actual bathtub to do a detox bath and exfoliating treatment. So when I need a little extra skin lift for my body, I wait until my skin is warm from the shower and then use the exfoliator square.

4. Stretchy cotton squares. I often feel dry after flying, and also

from traveling to the colder, drier Northeast. The cotton squares rehydrate my skin by doing a stretchy cotton mask (described in Chapter 3).

5. Tiny jar of raw honey. I use the honey for a quick face mask in the morning if my skin needs a little extra glow or moisture. It's also perfect for transporting local, raw honey if I want to add it to coffee or tea.

6. Small bottle of essential oils. Usually I bring lavender, chamomile, or a skincare blend. I use it for spot treatments or add it to my moisturizer. It also helps me relax after a long day on the road.

7. Tiny squares of luxurious soap. I cut a high quality, naturally scented soap from home into small chunks and place them in a plastic bag. That way, I don't have to carry a big hunk of messy, melty soap. I use it while I'm on the road so that I don't have to use the hotel soap which can be full of chemicals.

8. Two ounce container of coconut oil. I use coconut oil in the morning for oil pulling and then I also have a body moisturizer ready to go. I can also use it to remove eye makeup, as lip balm, or as a nighttime hand and cuticle treatment.

9. Tiny travel humidifier. Mine is made by Homedics. If you have dry skin and are in a winter climate, this little guy is a lifesaver.

Travel can be a time when you're prone to breakouts. Here are my favorite travel strategies to keep skin healthy and happy while on the road.

1. Grab a glass from your room and find the hotel ice machine to do an ice cube treatment.

2. Use fresh lemon wedges for a spot treatment. Find them in the hotel bar, at the airport, or at a restaurant or coffee shop.

3. At hotel check-in, ask for extra water. Keeping hydrated is key and as long as there's water in your room, you'll be re minded to keep drinking.

4. Use the bathroom shower to steam your clothes and add moisture to your room. Run the shower on hot, open the bathroom door, and let some of the steam into the air so you're not so dehydrated. Be sure to put down a towel and watch for any water on the floor. (I once slipped when I walked into the bathroom without seeing that I'd gotten water all over the floor!

Be sure to take your supplements while traveling. Keep powdered magnesium in your toiletry bag to take at night. Be sure to label and date everything so you don't confuse your clay with your gelatin, or any other of the odd things you might be taking.

I've only once had TSA ask about something in my bag. I was traveling with a few cups of Epsom salts and baking soda and the TSA guard was curious as to why I was carrying powder and crystals in bags. I have since stopped traveling with them, mainly because I've realized how hard it is to find time for a detox bath on the road. If needed, most grocery stores or drug stores have Epsom salts.

11

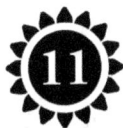

In Your New Skin

Though I've offered you an entire book full of skincare resources, I encourage you to continue your journey. Always continue investigating. Keep learning and growing to find exactly what your unique skin needs. Question everything you know, even this book, because that's how I figured it out. I came into my knowledge through a long journey of self-exploration which led to whole body healing and I want nothing less for you.

I continue to learn new things about my skin every day. Not everything is as it appears and our collective knowledge about skincare, wellness, and health is constantly evolving. Sometimes the most dramatic or counter-intuitive changes, like not washing your face, is exactly what your body needs. So be vigilant, be curious, and never settle, because acne is a symptom, not a trait. It is a message from your body that it needs your attention and now you have the tools to read that message.

Knowing what causes your breakouts gives you the power to manage them. Listen to your body with an open mind so that your skin doesn't become the carrier of your stress. Being informed, staying positive, and loving your skin creates a vibrant environment inside of your body. Remember that your skin works hard all day, every day to protect you. That it is constantly serving as your first layer of defense so appreciate it. Stay in tune with it. And take care of it with love.

If you find that you are still holding back, like I was, know that I understand how you feel. Beyond healing your skin, it takes courage and commitment to overcome the self-defeat that acne can instill in a person. But having come this far, you should feel proud. When you face the world, be the person you would be if you didn't have acne now. Because you are more than your skin. Don't hide your face, avoid your friends, or shut yourself in because the sooner that you let your inner light shine, the sooner your skin will begin to shine as well. Be the you who already has clear vibrant skin.

Resource Guide
& Further Reading

The goal of this book is to help you get immediate results without bogging you down in the details. However, every time I learned something about skin, I wanted to know why. Use the following resources to support your journey and deepen your understanding.

My Favorite Books:

A
Aromatherapy: Essential Oils for Vibrant Health & Beauty by Roberta Wilson

B
The Biology of Belief: Unleashing the Power of Consciousness, Matter & Miracles by Bruce H. Lipton, Ph.D.

C
Clean by Dr. Alejandro Junger, M.D. (This book is full of detailed instruction on how to conduct an elimination diet and includes specific recipes. It takes clean eating a step further by focusing on detoxification and alkaline foods.)

The Coconut Oil Miracle by Bruce Fife, C.N., N.D.

The Complete Book of Essential Oils & Aromatherapy by Valerie Ann Worwood

E

Earthing: The Most Important Health Discovery Ever? by Clinton Ober, Stephen T. Sinatra, M.D., and Martin Zucker

G

The Genie in Your Genes: Epigenetic Medicine and the New Biology of Intention by Dawson Church, Ph.D.

Grain Brain: The Surprising Truth about Wheat, Carbs, and Sugar—Your Brain's Silent Killers by David Perlmutter, M.D.

Gut and Psychology Syndrome: Natural Treatment for Autism, Dyspraxia, A.D.D., Dyslexia, A.D.H.D., Depression, Schizophrenia by Natasha Campbell-McBride, M.D.

H

The Hidden Messages in Water by Masaru Emoto

I

The Immune System Recovery Plan by Susan Blum, M.D., M.P.H. (This book is great specifically for autoimmune challenges.)

It Starts With Food: Discover the Whole30 and Change Your Life in Unexpected Ways by Dallas and Melissa Hartwig. (This was the first eating experiment I tried with amazing results.)

J

The Japanese Skincare Revolution: How to Have the Most Beautiful Skin of Your Life—At Any Age by Chizu Saeki

M
The Magic by Rhonda Byrne

Mind Over Medicine: Scientific Proof That You Can Heal Yourself by Lissa Rankin, M.D.

The Mindbody Prescription: Healing the Body, Healing the Pain by John E. Sarno, M.D.

N
A New Fighting Chance: Silver Solution by Gordon Pedersen, Ph.D.

Nourishing Traditions: The Cookbook that Challenges Politically Correct Nutrition and Diet Dictocrats by Sally Fallon

Nutrition and Physical Degeneration by Weston A. Price, D.D.S.

O
Oil Pulling Therapy, Detoxifying and Healing the Body through Oral Cleansing by Dr. Bruce Fife

P
The Paleo Approach, Reverse Autoimmune Disease and Heal Your Body by Sarah Ballantyne, Ph.D.

The Paleo Diet by Loren Cordain, Ph.D.

S
The Slow Down Diet, Eating for Pleasure, Energy, and Weight Loss by Marc David

T
The Tapping Solution: A Revolutionary System for Stress-Free Living by Nick Ortner

The Tapping Solution for Weight Loss & Body Confidence: A Woman's Guide to Stressing Less, Weighing Less, and Loving More by Jessica Ortner

Z

Zapped: Why Your Cell Phone Shouldn't Be Your Alarm Clock and 1,268 Ways to Outsmart the Hazards of Electronic Pollution by Ann Louise Gittleman

My Favorite Bloggers and Websites:

Juli Bauer of paleomg.com

Juil is my all-time favorite blogger. Juli's food is amazingly flavorful, her recipes are simple, and her sass and humor are a bonus. I have all of her cookbooks and especially love her latest, Juli Bauer's Paleo Cookbook.

Bill Stayley and Haley Mason of primalpalate.com

Bill and Haley have the most beautiful food photography, which definitely gets me in the cooking mood. I just picked up their latest book, Make It Paleo II, and it is incredible. They feature unique paleo foods that most others haven't tackled.

Brittany Angell of brittanyangell.com

Brittany is the author of Every Last Crumb: Paleo Bread and Beyond, a cookbook full of amazing paleo bread recipes. She's mastered the art of allergen-free baking and built an incredible niche with items like grain-free frosted (and sprinkled!) animal cookies, a paleo bloomin' onion, and even chocolate croissants, which used to be about the only thing you couldn't find grain-free. She's a phenom with specific and unique treats you can't find anywhere else. Not my everyday eating, but definitely my favorite for splurges!

Elana Amsterdam of elenaspantry.com
Simple, delicious and elegant, Elana uses very few ingredients in her foolproof recipes. I have all of her cookbooks and Paleo Cooking from Elana's Pantry is my favorite. I've fooled many family members with these healthy recipes.

Dave Aspery of bulletproofexec.com
Dave makes you question everything you thought you knew about health, and he has an awesome podcast. He supports a few high-end skincare products on his website that meet my skin standards, like amazing Alitura clay masks.

Tim Ferris of fourhourworkweek.com/blog
Tim is equal parts interesting and inspiring. He and Dave are my two favorite biohackers, life improvers, and status quo challengers. I own all three of Tim's incredible books. Top notch.

Mark Sisson of marksdailyapple.com
Mark is an original paleo guru and his blog is packed with great information. It's my go-to for detailed primal or paleo questions.

Dr. Joseph Mercola of mercola.com
Dr. Mercola is a leader in natural health. I go to his blog first for many issues.

Katie of wellnessmama.com
Katie's blog is full of great health, home, DIY, cleaning, clean skincare recipes and all around great information. I love it.

Heather Dessinger of mommypotamus.com
This blog is an amazing resource similar to wellnessmama.com. Heather has an amazing e-book called DIY Non-Toxic Cleaning Recipes that I highly recommend for switching out toxic ingredients in your home.

My Favorite Skincare Product Websites:

In case you are not ready to completely minimize your skincare route yet, here are some tried and true clean products available online.

Skin Apotheke at etsy.com/shop/Zria
I love this line of Aruveydic skincare.

Mad Hippie at madhippie.com
Clean and effective products. I especially love the vitamin C serum.

De La Terre Skincare at delaterreskincare.com
Plant-focused, super clean skincare line.

Tecniche skincare products at tecnicheskincare.com
Amazing line that work wonders for challenged and sensitive skin.

www.ingramcontent.com/pod-product-compliance
Lightning Source LLC
Chambersburg PA
CBHW052219270326
41931CB00011B/2411